T0304860

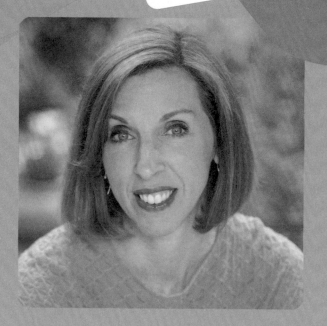

Dr Louise Newson

The Definitive Guide to the Perimenopause & Menopause

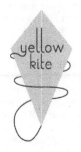

yellow
kite

First published in Great Britain in 2023 by Yellow Kite
An imprint of Hodder & Stoughton
An Hachette UK company

7

Copyright © Louise Newson Medical Writer Ltd 2023

The right of Dr Louise Newson to be identified as the Author
of the Work has been asserted by her in accordance with
the Copyright, Designs and Patents Act 1988.

Text design by Goldust Design

All rights reserved. No part of this publication may be reproduced, stored
in a retrieval system, or transmitted, in any form or by any means without
the prior written permission of the publisher, nor be otherwise circulated
in any form of binding or cover other than that in which it is published and
without a similar condition being imposed on the subsequent purchaser.

This book is intended as an accurate and informative guide. It is not
intended as a substitute for advice given to you by your doctor or other
healthcare professional. Before adopting any of the suggestions
in this book, we recommend that you consult with your chosen healthcare
professional as they are able to provide the necessary individualised care.
If you are receiving treatment for cancer, please do not embark on a new or
increased exercise regime unless this has been cleared by your healthcare
team. The author and publisher disclaim any liability incurred directly or
indirectly from the use of the information in this book by any person.

A CIP catalogue record for this title is available from the British Library

Hardback ISBN 978 1 399 70498 4
eBook ISBN 978 1 399 70500 4

Typeset in Charter by Hewer Text UK Ltd, Edinburgh
Printed and bound in Great Britain by Clays Ltd, Elcograf S.p.A.

Hodder & Stoughton policy is to use papers that are natural, renewable
and recyclable products and made from wood grown in sustainable
forests. The logging and manufacturing processes are expected to
conform to the environmental regulations of the country of origin.

Yellow Kite
Hodder & Stoughton Ltd
Carmelite House
50 Victoria Embankment
London EC4Y 0DZ

www.yellowkitebooks.co.uk

To my husband Paul.

Without his love, integrity and confidence then
I would be nothing.

Author's note

The guiding principle of this book – and my wider career – is to provide accurate and evidence based information about the perimenopause and menopause for all. Throughout, I refer to the menopause affecting women. 'Women', 'woman' and 'female' include anyone who experiences the perimenopause or menopause; I acknowledge a broader group of people who may identify as transgender, gender fluid, agender or non-binary, who may also experience the menopause.

Contents

Introduction   1

1   What Are Hormones – And
    Why Are They So Important?   7

2   Hormone Deficiency:
    Perimenopause and Menopause   31

3   Menopause and Family History   72

4   HRT: Everything You Need to Know   93

5   Mental Health and Menopause   135

6   Skin and Hair in the Menopause   160

7   Menopause in Younger People
    (Including Surgical Menopause)   179

8   Menopause and Cancer   202

9   Unseen and Unheard: Why the Menopause
    Conversation Must Be More Inclusive   236

10 Why Exercise Is One of the Best Forms of
    Medicine   257

11 Nutrition During the Perimenopause and
    Menopause   275

12 Menopause and Work   323

13 Looking to the Future   349

    Resources   357

    References   361

    Index   383

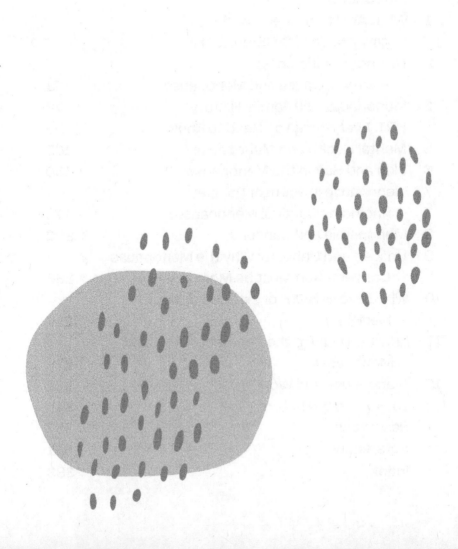

Introduction

It was late on a Friday afternoon when an email popped into my inbox.

The message was from a contact putting me in touch with Pete Smith, whose wife, Victoria, took her own life in 2021, after a two-year struggle with her mental health. A remarkable solicitor, described by her loved ones as calm, confident and the lynchpin of the family, Victoria was just fifty-one when she died.

In the months before her suicide, Victoria and Pete had asked those in charge of her care whether the change in her mental health was linked to the perimenopause – the time directly before the menopause when hormone fluctuations can affect mood. They asked whether Victoria's perimenopause could have been responsible for, or at least contributed to, her sudden mental illness when she had never previously experienced any such difficulties.

Pete says those questions were dismissed and, instead, Victoria was treated with a range of medication geared to treating clinical depression, starting with antidepressants and eventually lithium. A patient-safety investigation carried out by Victoria's local NHS trust after her death found that perimenopause could well have been one of the major factors they never seriously considered.

Pete was determined to raise awareness of the impact of peri-menopause and menopause, so no other family would have to go through what his did. So even though it was the end of another long working week, I knew I couldn't leave my desk without speaking to him. I picked up the phone and dialled his number and, if I'm honest, I didn't really know what I was going to say. What *can* you say to someone who has lost their wife in such awful circumstances?

Pete answered, and I was immediately struck with how strong and articulate he was. With a background in construction, he was the first to admit that menopause wasn't exactly the usual topic of conversation for him, but such was his determination that more people were informed about perimenopause and menopause that this didn't matter.

Like Pete, I too have a desire to raise awareness and help others: it is precisely the reason I have written this book. As a menopause specialist and GP, every year I see hundreds of women who are struggling with menopause, and thousands more reach out on social media looking for advice on symptoms like anxiety, fatigue and physical aches and pains that have impacted their relationships, social lives, confidence and careers.

The lack of knowledge and recognition of the impact of hormones on our physical and mental health (among women and healthcare professionals alike), scant research on women's health issues and confusion over treatments mean that many women are missing out on the support they need.

When the doors of my dedicated menopause clinic opened in 2018, I couldn't have predicted the surge of demand but, after hundreds of years, menopause is finally moving more into the mainstream.

And it's about time, too. Some 1.2 billion women worldwide are currently going through menopause. What was once a secretive issue that women barely spoke about even with their own daughters or close friends is now the term on everyone's lips, within families and right through to the boardroom.

With this explosion of interest comes the need for clear, practical information and advice. That's why I wanted this book to be a more detailed, deeper dive into menopause than anything I've ever done before.

In these pages are four key elements:

1. **The essentials**: must-know information that is evidence-based and accessible.
2. **Exclusive research**: for the purposes of this book, I have conducted surveys among women on everything from careers and relationships to mental health and will be sharing the findings here.
3. **Common questions answered**: I'll be using my experiences as both a doctor and a menopausal woman to make sure every page of this book answers your key questions.
4. **Expert views**: a panel of experts in fields including neurology, nutrition and psychology. In my working life, I am privileged to work with numerous professionals who make an incredible difference to women's lives, and throughout the book are their contributions on everything from mental health to nutrition. There are contributions from fitness guru Joe Wicks on exercise, renowned psychotherapist Julia Samuel on relationships, consultant dermatologist Sajjad Rajpar on hair and skincare, to name but a few.

I was also determined that this book should shine a light on the issues that are all too often overlooked when it comes to good menopause care. Issues like inequality of care for women from minority communities and early menopause, plus coping with menopause alongside other conditions, including cancer.

It's my wish that every woman who reads this book will have the information she needs to thrive during her menopause, and that loved ones and colleagues will get what they need in order to offer practical support.

How to use this book

This book is designed to be read however you want to. You can choose to read it from cover to cover to get a complete overview, or just dip in and out and look at the parts that are most relevant to you (there are sections on menopause and the workplace, relationships, family history, through to diet and exercise). However, whatever your reason for picking up this book, I'd advise that you read Chapters 1 and 2, which look at hormones, why they are so important for women's health, symptoms of perimenopause and menopause and the treatments that can help.

Menopause is anything but one size fits all, and your experience can differ from your relatives' and friends'. You might have terrible hot flushes, or you might never have a single one, for example. The start of each chapter clearly sets out four key things you will learn, while threaded throughout are 'timeouts', designed to help you get the most out of each section by posing key questions, encouraging you to think about the information *you* need to help you deal with your own particular symptoms and how you can advocate for yourself.

Read at your own pace, so you can absorb the information and use the timeouts and case studies as your time to reflect. Remember, this isn't a race – this is a resource to use how you want to. If you find it easier to read a few pages at a time in the bath or keep a copy by your bedside, then great. Or if, like me, you are a morning person and would better absorb information by flicking through at the weekend over your first coffee of the day, then go for it. It's completely up to you. Either way, I will be touching on some potentially personal and difficult subjects, so take a break when you need to – but remember how much better informed and positive you'll feel by the end of the book.

Now let's begin.

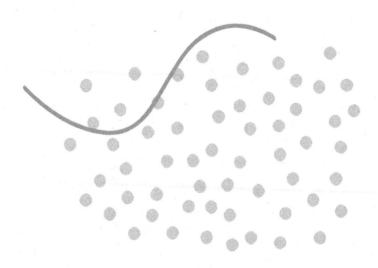

1

What Are Hormones – And Why Are They So Important?

Four things you will learn in this chapter:

1. What hormones are and why we need them

2. All about oestrogen, and the other key hormones

3. How hormones play a part during significant points in our lives, from PMS to pregnancy and post-birth

4. What happens when hormone levels fluctuate and fall

'Is it your hormones, dear?'

How many women have been on the receiving end of a tone-deaf statement like this when they've dared to show emotion or said something the other person hasn't agreed with?

Let's face it – our hormones do carry the can for changes to our physical and mental health. Slamming doors during your teenage years? That'll be your hormones. Feeling weepy, upset or just downright angry around the time your period is due? Hormones again. And many women with children will recall ghastly morning sickness during pregnancy or crashing moods in the days after giving birth. That's right, it's all down to hormones.

After each of my three children was born, I felt tearful, melancholy and low in my mood. I also experienced dreadful night sweats, terrible joint pains, crippling migraines and urinary symptoms, but naively thought these were all related to the tiredness you experience when having a baby. I just didn't think they were due to the rapid drop in hormone levels that had occurred. Everyone always talks about 'baby blues' without offering much – if any – help regarding actual treatment. I often wonder now how I would have felt if someone had given me some hormones to top up my very low levels.

But what about the good work that hormones do inside our bodies? And while we are on the subject, what exactly are hormones, anyway?

If you're picking up a book about the menopause, then it's probably safe to say you'll have heard of oestrogen, a key hormone in a woman's life. But a deeper understanding of the role of oestrogen and other hormones will help you to appreciate just how much falling levels affect you during perimenopause and menopause.

First, though, let's take a look at the role of hormones in supporting overall health and wellbeing.

Timeout #1: Hormones

Take a few minutes to consider what you may already know about hormones, the menopause and your overall health:

- How many hormones can you name?
- Where in the body are they produced?
- At what key events during a woman's life do hormones come into play?

Hormones explained

Simply put, hormones are chemical messengers found through-out your body to tell it what to do, and when. They are involved in your growth and development, metabolism, emotions, sexual and reproductive function, sleep and blood pressure. They help you fall in love, bond with offspring, power you to the finish line and make you feel happy, sad, furious and everything in between.

Hormones originate in your endocrine system – a network of organs containing glands that create and release them into your bloodstream. They then travel towards all your organs and tissues, where receptors in your cells recognise and respond to them.

Your endocrine system, and the hormones it produces, helps your bodies to maintain homeostasis – a constant internal envir-onment in response to internal and external changes – and to function properly. Compared to your nervous system, which uses not only chemicals but also electrical currents to help all parts of your body to communicate with each other, hormones are much slower and act over a longer period, sometimes years.

Endocrine glands are located throughout your body and include the following:

- **The hypothalamus:** located in your brain, the hypothalamus is a bit like the powerhouse of the endocrine system, linking your endocrine and nervous systems together.
- **Pituitary gland:** a pea-sized gland located at the base of your brain, the pituitary gland receives signals and secretes hormones from your hypothalamus and produces its own hormones.
- **Pineal gland:** located deep in your brain, this gland produces melatonin, a hormone that helps to regulate your wake–sleep cycle.
- **Thyroid gland:** a butterfly-shaped gland found at the base of your neck; thyroid hormones made here help to regulate your metabolism.
- **Parathyroid glands:** these four glands, found just behind your thyroid, secrete hormones to help your body maintain adequate calcium stores in your bloodstream to protect bone health.
- **Adrenal glands:** small, triangular-shaped glands located on top of both kidneys, these produce hormones in response to stress and help to regulate blood glucose and metabolism.
- **Pancreas:** situated in your upper abdomen behind your stomach and in front of your spine, the pancreas produces glucagon and insulin – hormones that help to regulate blood sugar.
- **Ovaries:** these are two small, oval-shaped organs in your pelvis located on either side of your uterus (womb). The ovaries produce the hormones oestrogen and progesterone

(I will be going into much more detail about the roles of your ovaries, oestrogen and progesterone). They also produce testosterone, another hormone.

Spotlight on oestrogen

Oestrogen is central to the development and functioning of your reproductive system, and the development of female characteristics, such as breasts. It also plays important roles in bone health, memory and cognition and cardiovascular health; in fact, there are oestrogen receptors in cells throughout your body.

Oestrogen is actually an umbrella term for three types:

- **Oestradiol**: the main form of oestrogen in your body during your reproductive years
- **Oestrone**: the main form of oestrogen that your body makes after menopause
- **Oestriol**: the main form of oestrogen during pregnancy

Chiefly made in the ovaries, but also in small amounts in the adrenal glands, oestrogen regulates the menstrual cycle – the process by which the body prepares for possible pregnancy. Every month, one of the ovaries releases an egg (known as ovulation). At the same time, hormonal changes prepare the uterus for pregnancy. If the egg isn't fertilised by a sperm, the lining of the uterus sheds through the vagina – and what we know as a period happens.

However, it is the effects of oestradiol on your immune cells that is the most important and relevant when it comes to your health. All your different immune cells have receptors for oestradiol on them and when it stimulates them, these cells can increase in number, be genetically reprogrammed and also change their function.

Research has shown that low oestradiol levels can lead to more inflammation in the body, whereas your immune cells work optimally when oestradiol levels are adequate. More inflammation leads to an increased risk of numerous conditions, including cardiovascular disease, osteoporosis and cancer. Even Alzheimer's disease, osteoporosis and clinical depression are considered to be inflammatory diseases.

When your immune system is not working optimally and there is more inflammation in your body, you age faster and the risk of disease increases. This process is often referred to as 'inflammageing'.

Menopause leads to accelerated inflammageing in your body, due to the low hormone levels that occur. A healthy lifestyle is also important in reducing inflammation.

Other important hormones you need to know about

Oestrogen is the main hormone we talk about during perimenopause and menopause, but there are a number of others you'll hear mentioned when it comes to discussing symptoms, tests and treatments.

Follicle-stimulating hormone (FSH)

This is released from your pituitary gland during menstruation and it stimulates your ovaries to produce oestrogen.

Luteinising hormone (LH)

LH is released from your pituitary gland at ovulation and causes your ovary to release an egg during ovulation.

Progesterone

Progesterone is another female hormone. Made in your ovaries, it works in your body to balance the effects of oestrogen and is often referred to as the relaxing hormone. Progesterone is produced after ovulation and dominates the second half of the menstrual cycle (luteal phase). Progesterone's main role is to control the build-up of your endometrium (uterine lining) and help maintain and mature it if there is a pregnancy.

Testosterone

An important sex hormone for both men and women (although women have much lower levels), this is produced by your ovaries and adrenal glands. Testosterone can work to maintain muscle and bone strength, enhance your sex drive and can help with your overall sense of wellbeing and zest for life.[1] Many women find that it can improve mood and stamina, as well as reducing brain fog and improving memory.

So as we now know, hormones are incredibly important for the functioning of your physical and mental health and maintaining homeostasis. But at different times of your life, your body creates and uses different amounts of hormones. And these hormonal upheavals can leave us feeling off balance, both physically and emotionally.

Premenstrual syndrome (PMS)

....

It's a familiar feeling many of us get in the run-up to our periods that we can't quite put our finger on.

You might feel overwhelmed, teary, anxious ... Or perhaps you find yourself on the other end of the mood spectrum – snapping at others, feeling irritated or angry. Maybe you notice physical symptoms, such as tender or heavy breasts, or you might be a bit more accident-prone than usual. Often, these feelings can be downplayed or dismissed as something women have to put up with each month – but for some, they can have a real impact.

PMS is when you have distressing symptoms in the days or even weeks leading up to starting your period. It encompasses an array of psychological and physical symptoms (see p. 15) and is identified when these occur, and have a negative impact, during the luteal phase of your menstrual cycle – between ovulation (normally mid-cycle, around day 14) and starting your period (usually around day 28).

Although the average length of the menstrual cycle is twenty-eight days, it can vary greatly from person to person, and you may find the length of your cycle varies from month to month.

Why does PMS happen?

Although the precise causes of PMS have yet to be identified (there may be a genetic susceptibility for some women), there is compelling evidence to suggest that symptoms are directly related to the body's response to fluctuations in hormone levels in the monthly cycle.[2]

And it's worth pointing out that PMS is not usually seen in young girls who have not started their periods, during pregnancy

14

or post-menopause in most women. PMS appears to begin, or increase in severity, at times of marked hormonal change, such as in puberty (even before the first period happens), starting or stopping the oral contraceptive pill, after pregnancy and during the perimenopause.

What sort of symptoms occur?

More than 150 symptoms of PMS have been identified, and these are usually grouped into psychological and behavioural ones and physical ones.

Common psychological and behavioural symptoms:

- Mood swings
- Depression
- Tiredness, fatigue or lethargy
- Anxiety
- A feeling of a loss of control

- Irritability
- Aggression
- Anger
- Disordered sleep
- Food cravings

Common physical symptoms:

- Breast tenderness (mastalgia)
- Bloating

- Clumsiness
- Headaches

All the above are similar to perimenopausal and menopausal symptoms – not surprising, as the underlying cause is the same (low hormone levels). On the whole, the majority of women will experience only a few of these symptoms; usually, one or two may be dominant and each can vary in severity, both during a cycle and from one cycle to another. New symptoms may present at any time during a woman's experience of PMS, and symptoms may be experienced continuously from ovulation to menstruation, for just the seven days before menstruation, at ovulation for three or four days, and/or just prior to menstruation. In some cases, you might not experience relief from symptoms until the day of your period's heaviest flow.

CASE STUDY: PMS – SARAH'S STORY

Sarah first realised she was affected by PMS in her late teens. Now in her forties, and although not yet perimenopausal, she is already planning to monitor any changes in her PMS, which can be an early sign of perimenopause:

'I started my periods in my final year of primary school.

'Being the youngest and the only girl in my family, I remember feeling pretty embarrassed and confused. Luckily, my teacher was really lovely and supportive, and she gave me a sanitary towel from her handbag and talked me through how to use it.

'I suppose I was what some people would define as a "moody teen", although I really hate that label. I was embarrassed at my developing body and would hide myself in big sweatshirts or hooded tops (it was the early 1990s, when grunge was all the rage, so at least it was the fashion).

'It was when I had my first serious boyfriend in my late teens that I really noticed that my moods would coincide with my periods. In the run-up, I would become teary and withdrawn or get instantly irritated by a comment that probably wouldn't bother me at other times of the month.

'My then boyfriend would comment on how it was hard to plan days out when I was due on my period because the day would always end in an argument, or I'd feel nervous and uncomfortable trying somewhere new. At the time, I lived with three other girls and, bar cramps and back pain, none of them seemed to be affected in the way I was by PMS.

'When I had my first child in my early thirties, my mood was very low, but I never really connected that with hormones and, once my periods started again, I was back in the familiar territory of PMS.

'While I don't view my PMS as being at the severe end – I can still work and go out – there are things I do to try to mitigate my symptoms. I find being upfront with people helps – my kids know that there are times of the month when Mummy doesn't feel 100 per cent, and I try to schedule work deadlines at different times of the month (though that's not always possible).

'I'm not quite at the perimenopause stage yet, but I've read up on the various symptoms and have resolved to keep a close eye on my PMS to see if anything changes.'

Premenstrual dysphoric disorder (PMDD)

This term is becoming increasingly used to describe a very severe version of a core premenstrual disorder that can be extremely distressing. The criteria for diagnosing PMDD are very stringent and always include mood-related symptoms. The symptoms must occur in the luteal phase, and they must be severe enough to disrupt your day-to-day life.

How many people are affected by PMS and PMDD?

PMS can occur in any woman during her child-bearing years. Studies have shown that about 80–90 per cent of women manifest at least one of the PMS symptoms; however, in about 3 per cent of women they are severe enough to affect their activities and social communications.[3] It can have a significant and detrimental effect on their quality of life, impacting not only themselves, but their whole network of relationships – including partners, children, relatives, friends and work colleagues. And the fluctuating nature of symptoms can be unsettling for all involved.

Getting a diagnosis

There is no blood test to confirm PMS or PMDD, so keeping a diary of the timing and impact of symptoms on everyday activities is crucial in reaching a diagnosis.

I would advise keeping a diary for a minimum of two cycles and recording symptoms as they happen, while they are fresh in your mind, rather than relying on memory. And the good news is that charts and questionnaires have been developed for this purpose.

A questionnaire called the DRSP (Daily Record of Severity of Problems) is sometimes used by healthcare professionals, so you may be asked to fill this out. You can also download a chart from the National Association for Premenstrual Syndrome (NAPS) website, while the US-based International Association for Premenstrual Disorders has a symptom tracker (see Resources, p. 357 for both). Alternatively, some women find using a period-tracking app useful for logging symptoms and monitoring how they change over the course of a cycle. My balance menopause app (the only menopause app certified by ORCHA – Organisation for the Review of Care and Health Apps; see Resources, p. 357) also allows you to log and track your periods and symptoms and provides your clinician with a health report, which can be used to help both diagnose and treat your PMS.

If a symptom diary proves inconclusive, an alternative way of diagnosing PMS or PMDD is to temporarily shut off your ovaries using medication. Gonadotropin-releasing hormone (GnRH) analogues are a group of drugs that are modified versions of a naturally occurring hormone in your body, which helps to control your menstrual cycle. Shutting down your body's production of oestrogen and progesterone for three months using a GnRH analogue will usually stop your menstrual cycle occurring and should, in theory, reduce or stop PMS symptoms. If this does not happen, then other causes should be considered.

Hormonal treatment for PMS and PMDD

HRT should be considered first choice treatment for these hormonal depressions. The oestrogen treatment is given with progesterone that is usually taken for 2 weeks per month, and this pattern will trigger a monthly bleeding cycle. The progesterone helps keep the womb lining thin and healthy. If you have not had a hysterectomy, you could alternatively have the Mirena coil fitted, which releases a type of progesterone. You may also be offered testosterone as this can improve mood, energy levels and libido.

The use of moderately high doses of transdermal oestrogen (taken through the skin in a patch, gel or spray) is often recommended to suppress ovulation in women with PMS and PMDD.

Common doses would be 200mcg patches (twice weekly) or 4mg daily if oestrogen gel. This approach often balances out the profoundly fluctuating oestrogen levels to help stabilise your body's reaction to the hormones and lessen symptoms.

In severe cases of PMS, the use of GNRH analogues are sometimes used. This is a hormone medication that 'switches off' the ovaries altogether, usually given with add back HRT to prevent the associated risks from a lack of hormones and improve future health. This medication tends to be recommended when other treatments have been unsuccessful.

EXPERT VIEW
Seeking help for PMS – Dr Hannah Ward,
GP and menopause specialist

Dr Hannah works within my clinic, as well as in general practice. Her interest in the menopause and HRT was ignited following her own hormonal struggles after the birth of her children, and she now spends much of her time in general practice helping women to recognise the effects of hormones on their physical and mental health.

It can be common for women to downplay PMS, but severe symptoms can really impact your life.

Another problem is that medics aren't taught enough about hormones and the problems that can arise when there is a hormonal imbalance. I know when I first started as a GP, I didn't really understand how crucial it was to balance hormones.

When it comes to worsening symptoms of PMS during peri-menopause, I always say to my patients that it's like going through puberty in reverse. Those mood swings and hormone fluctuations that happened at that stage can return during peri-menopause, and that can exacerbate PMS.

Knowledge is power

Increasingly, I'm seeing younger women in their twenties and late teens using apps to track their menstrual cycle, which I think is a very positive thing. When I think back to my teenage years, no one ever really told me about the menstrual cycle and how oestrogen and our periods affect us. If you think that you might be experiencing PMS, start tracking your cycle and identify any common symptoms. When you are aware of issues, you can consider what you can do about tackling them.

Look at diet and lifestyle

While balanced diet won't 'cure' moderate to severe PMS, it can certainly help symptoms.

For example, try to avoid white refined carbohydrates, found in foods like white bread, because they can cause a rapid release of blood glucose, which can, in turn, contribute to weight gain and impact mood swings.

Some studies suggest B vitamins, specifically B6, can help with PMS-related depression and generalised symptoms.

And watch your alcohol and caffeine intake: both can increase anxiety.

See a healthcare professional if you are struggling

A lot of women will see their symptoms as 'just' PMS. But if your life is being affected by your symptoms, see a healthcare professional to talk about any potential treatments.

As Dr Louise suggests, track your symptoms and (as mentioned above) your periods and bring that information along to your appointment. Think about the symptom/s that affect you the most and be sure to mention those. Talk to your healthcare professional about the possibility of taking hormones too.

Hormones at play during pregnancy

Our bodies go through incredible changes during pregnancy, with hormones taking centre stage in maintaining pregnancy and preparing the body for birth. Let's look at the key hormones and the parts they play.

Oestrogen

As we know, oestrogen is produced in your ovaries, but in pregnancy it is also produced by the placenta, an organ that develops in your uterus during pregnancy as a source of oxygen and nutrients for the growing foetus. Oestrogen helps to maintain a healthy pregnancy, and is involved in the development of female sexual traits in a female foetus.

Progesterone

Sometimes referred to as the pregnancy hormone, progesterone stimulates the thickening of your uterine lining for implantation of a fertilised egg. It supports the early stages of pregnancy, helps to establish the placenta and is involved with strengthening pelvic-floor muscles in the latter stages of pregnancy, ready for labour.

Human chorionic gonadotropin hormone (hCG)

Levels of hCG, a hormone only made during pregnancy in the placenta, peak in the first trimester and are thought to play a part in morning sickness. I was fortunate, as I only had mild morning sickness, which was worst during the first three months of my first pregnancy. It was enough to make me feel really uncomfortable, and I often struggled at work because during consultations with patients I would sometimes have an urge to retch and vomit, which was really unpleasant. When I was doing obstetrics and gynaecology as part of my GP training, I would often admit women into hospital with severe morning sickness and they required an intravenous drip of fluid and several nights in hospital. Some even had symptoms throughout their entire pregnancies and, all too often, felt the seriousness of these was underestimated by others.

Human placental lactogen (hPL)

Also known as human chorionic somatomammotropin, hPL is made by the placenta during pregnancy; it provides nutrition to the growing foetus and stimulates milk glands in the breasts ready for breastfeeding.

Oxytocin

Produced in your hypothalamus and secreted by your pituitary gland, oxytocin encourages contractions during labour and helps with bleeding after birth. Also known as the cuddle hormone, oxytocin helps to foster bonding with your baby after birth and with milk production.

Prolactin

Produced in your pituitary gland, prolactin helps with milk production (the clue is in the name) and, similar to oxytocin, this hormone also helps with bonding.

Hormones after having a baby

I've never been a fan of the term 'baby blues'. It sounds too fluffy and does little to reflect the reality of being a new parent and the hormonal upheaval that comes with it.

I remember like it was yesterday the weight of responsibility I felt when we brought our eldest daughter, Jess, home from the hospital. There we were, two doctors with years of training in our specialisms. But years in both medical school and practice really didn't prepare me for those early days and weeks after having a baby, or for the attendant hormone crash. I soon felt low in my mood, more irritable and tearful at times. I had very little patience and was often very short-tempered. I experienced both discomfort and some increased frequency in passing urine and had many nights when I woke up drenched with sweat, but many people told me this was normal when breastfeeding, and I did not, at any stage, attribute the symptoms to my low hormone levels. Instead, I assumed many of these feelings and symptoms were due to being tired from having recently had a baby.

In the immediate days after giving birth, you may find your mood is very low. I remember thinking how this was supposed to be the absolute happiest time of my life, yet I couldn't stop crying. Welcome to the so-called baby blues. Other symptoms can include:

- feeling emotional (this could include bursting into tears for no apparent reason)
- irritability
- anxiety
- feeling restless[4]

I remember after Jess was born alternating between the urge to just shut myself away and a restless feeling of wanting to go on long walks to clear my head.

The stream of visitors you have when your first baby is born can be overwhelming and I found it quite difficult to cope with. And while we are on the subject, please, please don't turn up at the home of a woman who has just given birth and expect them to make you a cup of tea or some lunch. Offer to bring food with you, put some laundry on, do the vacuuming . . . Think of yourself as less of a visitor and more of a helper. Asking a simple question like, 'What can I do to help?' is incredibly important and often the best form of support you can provide.

Why does this hormonal upheaval happen?

Right after delivery of the baby and placenta, oestrogen and progesterone – having worked so hard to protect the foetus and prepare the mother for birth – plummet, returning to pre-pregnancy levels, within twenty-four hours, it is thought. The baby is here, so their work is done, the body says. In turn, levels of oxytocin and prolactin surge, designed to help with bonding and milk production, but they too will start to level off in the days after giving birth.

And how long does the upheaval last?

It's important to remember that the feelings you can experience after your baby is born are completely normal, but they should be temporary and should subside about two weeks after giving birth.

Postnatal depression (PND)

There's no getting around it: having a young baby can be very tough. Really tough. Caring for a little human who relies on you for everything, getting back to physical health after giving birth and the general juggling of life, relationships and other caring responsibilities mean you might not feel like 'you' for some time after the birth. But while baby-blues-type symptoms lessen around two weeks after the birth, you should be vigilant about postnatal depression.

One of my jobs as a GP was carrying out the six-week postnatal check – an appointment where I would check in on the physical and mental wellbeing of a new mother six to eight weeks after giving birth. This appointment is often a crucial touchpoint for new mothers to address any health issues postbirth. I remember clearly how while many mothers would be forthcoming about any physical issues, some would shake their heads or clam up when I asked if they were struggling with their mental health. PND frequently goes unrecognised because many women regard this degree of depression and exhaustion as a normal consequence of looking after a new baby. And those who are struggling with upsetting thoughts, especially those of harm, often will not confide in another person.

Yet about one in ten women will experience PND in the year after giving birth. Often, the symptoms were evident to me as a healthcare professional, but some mothers either felt it wasn't worth mentioning, were unduly worried about 'wasting' my time or they simply didn't know the common signs of PND or recognise it in themselves.

What are the symptoms?

According to the charity PANDAS Foundation (PND Awareness and Support; see Resources, p. 360), symptoms can include the following:

- Low mood and persistent sadness
- Lack of energy
- Difficulty bonding with baby
- Over- and undereating for comfort
- Frightening and intrusive thoughts
- Lack of enjoyment and loss of interest in the wider world
- Trouble sleeping at night and feeling sleepy during the day
- Withdrawing from contact with other people
- Lack of concentration and difficulty making decisions

Why does it happen?

It is very likely that the root cause of postnatal depression is the sudden decrease in hormones (particularly oestrogen) that occurs after delivery. PND can be more severe and more prolonged in women who breastfeed, as this suppresses oestrogen levels further.

There are many different treatments for PND, often including antidepressants and psychological treatments. However, many clinicians still do not offer or give hormones that would likely help, even though they will treat the underlying cause. This is often because giving replacement hormones is not discussed in management guidelines for PND. Clearly more work and research really needs to be done in this area.

CASE STUDY: PND – LUCY'S STORY

Lucy was ecstatic when she found out she was pregnant with her youngest child, Thomas (now five), but having a second baby brought mental-health challenges.

'I thought I was a pro at the pregnancy and childbirth game when I was pregnant with my second. I bought up all the snacks and remedies that had got me through the awful morning sickness that had been a constant companion during my first pregnancy. (It was so bad first time around that I cried tears of relief back on the ward after having my baby, when I realised that for the first time in months I didn't feel nauseous.)

'Second time around, I asked for and accepted offers of help where possible, because I knew I had to conserve my energy, especially with a toddler to look after. Even giving birth second time around, I felt more in control and assertive about following the wishes recorded in my birth plan.

'My son Thomas was born during a particularly cold February, so those early weeks were mainly spent indoors, aside from the visit to the baby weigh-in clinic at our local health centre or going to the odd parent-and-baby class.

'I'd had the "baby blues" with my eldest, but with my second, when that familiar weepy feeling came over me in the days after the birth it hit me much harder. I told myself it was just my hormones, and that things would settle down.

'As the weather got milder and life settled into a pattern, my mood was still quite flat, so I resolved to get out and start seeing people again. I signed up to every class possible: baby yoga, singing, music and movement, baby massage – you name it, I tried it. And I filled the rest of the day going on long walks or looking around the shops. Deep down, I craved noise and activity because I didn't want to be alone with my own thoughts.

'Looking back, I can see how my anxiety manifested itself. If I missed a slot for a class, I would agonise about Thomas's development. If I didn't feel part of the "mum gang" at a class, I would worry I had said the wrong thing. I would obsess over health issues and turn to parenting websites for advice and validation, instead of speaking to my own health visitor or family doctor. I was always too restless to read or sit through an episode of a TV programme. I'd put it down to the tiredness I constantly felt, or the fact that the baby needed me or we had somewhere to be.

'No matter how I filled my days, I felt hollow, but I still thought it was the tiredness of having two children under three. Things came to a head when I arrived at the children's centre to find they'd overbooked a session. I took it so personally and broke down in tears of frustration. Luckily, one of the health visitors was on site and took me into a side room. It sounds like a cliché, but all it took was someone to look me in the eye and ask if I was ok to realise no, I absolutely wasn't.

'A family-doctor appointment followed and a diagnosis of PND was made and I was able to access help. At that point, my son was just shy of a year, so I'd been carrying this around for months. Looking back, I wish I'd kept a little sort of checklist of symptoms to keep an eye on. I think if I had, I would have realised when baby blues and tiredness turned into PND.'

SURVEY: HOW MUCH DO YOU KNOW ABOUT HORMONES?

In November 2022, I launched a wide-ranging survey, the findings of which are woven throughout this book.

The response was truly overwhelming: within days, almost 6,000 women had shared their experiences, their stories and their views.

One of the topics covered in the survey was knowledge of hormones.

Very encouragingly, 99 per cent of respondents said they had heard of oestrogen, 98 per cent had heard of progesterone and 94 per cent had heard of testosterone.

Other hormones were less familiar; 54 per cent had heard of follicle-stimulating hormone (FSH), and 39 per cent had heard of luteinising hormone.

One in 10 (11 per cent) of respondents had a diagnosis of PMS, 1 per cent PMDD and one in eight (12 per cent) had had a diagnosis of postnatal depression.

Many respondents laid bare how hormonal changes had affected their physical and mental health.

'For two weeks of the month I was a different person; crying spells, loneliness, depression, basically feeling horrendous,' said one.

We have covered the role of hormones in conditions like PMS and PMDD and, if you have had children, how hormones can affect you during pregnancy and after giving birth. So you may well think you've had enough of the hormonal rollercoaster to last a lifetime – but there are two more hormonal shifts on the horizon: the perimenopause, followed by the menopause. The next chapter covers everything you need to know about these, from symptoms through to getting a diagnosis.

2

Hormone Deficiency: Perimenopause and Menopause

Four things you will learn in this chapter:

1. From head to toe – what happens when hormone levels fall

2. How to tell if you are perimenopausal or menopausal

3. Why tracking symptoms is essential for a correct diagnosis

4. Increased knowledge of the range of menopausal symptoms

A few years ago, when I was working in general practice, a woman in her mid-forties came to see me in clinic. Let's call her Jo.

Jo had been a patient at the surgery for some years, but not one we saw regularly. She had a successful career, was in a stable, loving relationship, ate well, exercised regularly and was generally in good health. Despite this, she was struggling.

She felt tired all the time, her concentration wavered and, for some unknown reason, her knees really hurt. Her initial thought was that she might be lacking in vitamins, so she went out and bought some expensive supplements. She took them for a few months in the hope of an improvement, but nothing changed.

During Jo's appointment, we talked about her medical history; she had a clean bill of health. When I asked her which symptom concerned her the most, she said it was the issue with concentration. She was having to write more things down and would lose her train of thought midway through a phone call – and she was worried colleagues had started to notice. Deep down, Jo admitted, she was worried about her memory in the long term.

I then asked about her periods. She paused, started counting on her fingers and shrugged.

'I suppose I've not had one for about four or five months.'

I had already started to specialise in the menopause at that stage, so for me, the diagnosis was pretty clear. I explained that based on her age, her symptoms and the fact she hadn't had a period in several months, Jo was perimenopausal.

When I delivered the news, she looked instantly relieved. But then the relief turned to a familiar look of bemusement that I'd seen in numerous patients before, and many since.

'But I can't be!' she exclaimed. 'I haven't had a single hot flush. And besides, I'm only in my forties.'

Jo's symptoms weren't particularly rare or numerous, nor was her diagnosis difficult – in fact, it was pretty much textbook. But I'm sharing this story because it lays bare the perception issue that has plagued menopause care for decades. The perception that the menopause only happens to women of a 'certain age'. The perception that because the menopause is often natural, you trust your body and let nature take its course. The perception (from women) that the menopause isn't really something you want to bother your doctor about. And the perception that hot flushes are the only symptom.

Well, wrong, wrong, wrong – and wrong again.

Yet Jo is far from unusual in her thinking. In fact, I too didn't realise I was perimenopausal for several months. I know, I know. A menopause specialist who didn't recognise her own perimenopause. You couldn't make it up, could you? But the simple fact is that back when I was in my mid-forties, I didn't know what I know now. It took my then eleven-year-old daughter to give me the nudge I needed.

So let me take you back to 2015.

I was forty-five, working as a GP and raising three young daughters.

The changes were barely noticeable at first, but the cumulative effect left me feeling miserable, flat and, to put it mildly, shattered.

First, my PMS was worse than ever. I'd always suffered from mood changes and migraines in the run-up to my period, but now these seemed to happen more often and last longer.

I'd also started suffering from night sweats. I'd dread going to bed each evening, as I knew the chances that I would wake up in the middle of the night drenched in sweat were pretty high. On more than one occasion, these night sweats were so bad I mistakenly thought I'd wet myself. Every time, I felt so ashamed. I would often rush to the bathroom for a cool shower and change of pyjamas and would even sometimes wake my husband, Paul, so I could change the sheets. You can imagine how much laundry we did during those months.

All that nocturnal activity of waking up, showering, changing bedding and clothing meant I was turning up to my surgery feeling like I'd already worked a double night shift, and I lived in fear of making a mistake.

Looking back, I was so completely and utterly tired. It reminded me of the enveloping tiredness I'd experienced when I was heavily pregnant: the slow, wading-through-treacle feeling when even the act of getting out of bed in the morning felt like an uphill climb. Only this time, I wasn't pregnant.

At home, things started to slip. Any working parent knows the dance of getting everyone up and out of the door on time in the morning, the organisational skills needed to co-ordinate drop-offs and pick-ups to various clubs and social engagements. I was by no means supermum, but I could usually keep on top of things and make sure our daughters had everything they needed.

But I found that as the months dragged on, the more tired and tense I became and the less able I was to cope. I'd get easily irritated and snap at the children, and I lacked both the energy and the desire to do any of the fun family things we'd previously enjoyed. I'm the sort of person who is always on the go, but all I wanted to do when I got home from work was crawl into bed.

My marriage was affected, too. All the night sweats and tossing and turning didn't exactly scream romance and being so short-tempered meant I wasn't the easiest person to live with. Little things that wouldn't have bothered me before became big issues: even the sound of my husband's breathing annoyed me. I stopped seeing friends, using work as an excuse – and even missed some work functions as I had no interest in socialising. I stopped reading novels and found it too hard to concentrate on watching a film. Even cooking food (which I have always enjoyed) was laborious and difficult.

The fact is, I was running on empty.

In healthcare we often talk about resilience. Working in medicine and wider healthcare is an immensely rewarding career, but it can be tough on you emotionally. As a clinician, you have a duty to provide the best level of care for your patients. You are there for the celebratory moments when a scan comes back clear, or when a patient is finally allowed to be discharged and go home to their family. But there are also the times when you have to break bad news that no one wants to hear and be there to offer support and sometimes a shoulder to cry on.

Family doctors are there from cradle to grave. On any one day in my work in general practice I could be seeing a newborn baby, organising a referral for a patient with suspected cancer and discussing end-of-life care arrangements with the relatives of someone whose final wish is to die at home, surrounded by family.

As a doctor, you build up a second skin to deal with these highs and lows, allowing you to stay professional and continue going into work, day after day. And that second skin can carry you through difficult times in your personal life, too. I have always tried to be practical, looking for answers and solutions. But during those months in my mid-forties, it felt like I was out of resilience, energy, patience – and out of excuses.

I hadn't even considered the perimenopause. Part of me worried that my night sweats and fatigue might be a sign of something more serious, like lymphoma (a type of cancer), but instead of doing the sensible thing and booking an appointment with my doctor, I thought I'd give it a bit more time to see if the symptoms would settle down on their own.

Things came to a head one evening when, while making dinner, I experienced a hot flush for the very first time. At first, I thought it was the heat of the pan, but then I realised it was coming from *inside* of me, spreading from my chest to my neck and head. It only lasted for a few seconds, but it felt like for ever.

I put my hand on the counter to steady myself, and my daughter, Sophie, noticing something was wrong, looked up from her homework to ask why I was so hot and sweaty. In that moment, I felt embarrassed and confused, and I'm ashamed to say she got her head bitten off for that observation.

She then asked me why I had been so short-tempered with all the family over the preceding few months. She even asked if I was due a period, as some of her friends were (her words) 'quite stroppy' before their periods.

I tried to brush her questions off, but later that evening, when I was alone in the kitchen, I came to reflect on what she had said.

Why had it irked me so much? And come to think of it, when *was* I due my period? And then, like Jo in my consulting room a few years later, I sat at the kitchen table counting on my fingers and doing some mental maths.

It then dawned on me that it had been several months since my last period. What would cause my periods to be irregular or stop altogether? I definitely wasn't pregnant. So what were all the moods, the migraines, the night sweats and now my first ever hot flush all adding up to?

Perimenopause.

I don't want you to be like I was during those first months of my perimenopause: feeling tired, irritated, wondering what on earth was going on and putting off an appointment to see the doctor. And that is why we are now going to look at exactly what happens during the perimenopause and menopause, so you are informed.

Perimenopause

The clinical definition of the *menopause* is when you have not had a period for twelve consecutive months. The *perimenopause* is a time of transition directly before that, when hormone levels start to decline and menopausal symptoms start. Your periods may still be regular at this time or you may find that they have changed in nature or frequency (or both).

Let's look at some statistics to explain why the perimenopause happens:

- The menstrual cycle (as covered in the previous chapter) works to release a mature egg (ovulation) every month in preparation for possible fertilisation and pregnancy.
- Over her lifetime, a woman's ovaries will release about 500 mature eggs.
- Girls have about 2 million eggs at birth, reducing to about 400,000 by the time they reach adolescence. Fertility peaks between late teens and early thirties and, by the age of thirty-seven, women roughly have 25,000 eggs left.
- By the age of fifty-one (the average age of menopause in the UK), women have fewer than 1,000 eggs remaining.[5]

When the egg supply reduces, levels of the hormones oestrogen and progesterone fall, too. And when your hormones fluctuate and fall, all the systems that have relied on them start to feel their absence, triggering symptoms.

Timeout #1: Focus on periods

If you aren't yet in the menopause, take a few minutes to reflect:

- How often do you have periods? Do you keep track each month?
- Do you tend to be regular or irregular?
- Think about flow: are your periods heavy, light or have there been any changes recently?
- Have you noticed any PMS-like symptoms (see p. 15) in the run-up to your period?

When should I expect the perimenopause to happen?
As a general rule, the perimenopause begins in the early to mid-forties – though it can happen later or much earlier for reasons including genetics or due to surgery or treatment (we'll cover this in Chapters 7 and 8).

If I were to draw a graph charting your oestrogen levels through your teens and into your twenties, thirties and beyond, you would see that (in line with the falling off of your egg supply, as described above) they are usually at their highest in your late twenties to thirties, before starting to decline from your early forties onwards, then hitting an all-time low around the fifty mark.

The line from your forties into your fifties is not a smooth one, however. Rather, it is wiggly – because oestrogen levels can fluctuate, being lower one day and higher the next. And this is because ovarian function can also fluctuate during the perimenopause. Think of it as the time your ovaries are winding down.

So what do these fluctuations mean?

Some women might not have any symptoms, or will barely notice any, while others may be plagued with severe ones for months or even years. As with everything to do with perimenopause and menopause, it is an entirely unique experience.

Changes to your periods

For starters, your menstrual cycle will usually be affected. It might get longer or shorter; I went several months without a period, but you might find yours come closer together and are heavier than usual.

Changing oestrogen levels mean your ovaries may not release an egg as regularly as they used to. You may ovulate one month, and then not, and the quality of eggs also declines as you get older.

PMS

In addition to changing periods, you might find, like I did, that PMS-like symptoms such as mood changes and breast tenderness become more severe.

Studies have shown that PMS sufferers are twice as likely to experience hot flushes and mood swings in their perimenopause compared to women who do not have a history of PMS. So if you have been troubled by PMS throughout your life, this may be a predictor that you will experience unwanted symptoms during your perimenopause. Alternatively, women who may never have experienced noticeable PMS symptoms in the past may start struggling with them now.

Though in my experience they tend to be early indicators, perimenopause symptoms are not just limited to PMS and period changes.

The time has come: the menopause

It's common for women to positively dread their menopause. But I want to stress that it can be – and often is – a very positive and empowering experience.

As explained earlier, you are deemed to be 'in' the menopause when you haven't had a period for twelve months. If you are still having the odd period here and there, you are probably still peri-menopausal – remember, this stage can last for several years.

You might have a gut feeling that you are already menopausal, so the remainder of this chapter is all about setting out the myriad potential symptoms that can be experienced – and why. But please *don't panic*. You may not have a single symptom, or you might just have a handful. The best approach is to face it head on: understand the symptoms and the causes and recognise any changes in your body.

Timeout #2: Noticing anything different?

- If you've been tracking your periods, has it been twelve months or more since your last one?
- Have you noticed any other changes in your body or mood?
- Has anyone – friends, colleagues, partners – remarked on any differences in you lately?

Get tracking

You may have had a condition in the past where a healthcare professional has asked you to keep a symptom diary. This is to help pinpoint the scale and severity and spot any patterns, and it's really useful in making a diagnosis.

If you decide that you need help with your menopause symptoms, you may find your mind goes blank and you can't remember which bother you most, or how long they have been going on for. And that's where tracking them comes in. It's your aide-memoire for a health appointment, so you can focus on the conversation, rather than sit there racking your brain for times and dates.

How you record all this is up to you. You could grab a big sheet of paper, note it down on your phone or in a diary or use the symptom tracker on my balance app (see Resources, p. 357).

However you choose to do it, though, you'll need to record three key things:

- What symptom you have – be it physical or psychological
- How often it happens
- How severe it is

But how will you know which symptoms to record?

You have oestrogen receptors throughout your body and low levels of oestrogen can throw up an array of symptoms during the perimenopause and menopause, from the obvious and the well-known, like changes to periods or hot flushes, through to the downright baffling, such as bad breath, burning tongue and heart palpitations. Use this chapter as a chance to familiarise yourself with all of these, and, if you experience any of them, make a note of them via your chosen method.

Abdominal pain and other gastrointestinal symptoms

Some women find they develop intermittent stomach pains and other symptoms similar to irritable bowel syndrome, such as bloating, trapped wind, constipation or even diarrhoea.

Why does it happen?

Hormone receptors in your gastrointestinal (GI) system are sensitive to changes in oestrogen and progesterone levels. During the menstrual cycle, a rise in progesterone can slow down motility (the movement of food through the GI tract), leading to constipation, while rising oestrogen levels during ovulation also help food to pass through our GI tract. Often, symptoms like bloating, constipation and diarrhoea can occur during the

HORMONE DEFICIENCY: PERIMENOPAUSE AND MENOPAUSE

perimenopause in response to fluctuating hormones. Declining oestrogen can also impact on the hormones cortisol and adrenaline, which can play important roles in your digestive process.

Altered sense of smell and taste

One of the most surprising symptoms is an altered sense of smell. You might find you can't smell things as keenly as you used to, this sense might be heightened or there may even be certain smells – such as perfumes and cleaning products – you just can't stand any more. This can then affect your sense of taste, too.

Why does it happen?

Oestrogen can affect the pathways in your brain that control your sense of smell and taste. You might find that the changes only last for a few days, or longer.

As a side note, a heightened sense of smell is actually a fairly common occurrence in pregnancy, too. I remember when I was pregnant wanting to treat myself to something special, so I decided to splash out on a gorgeous perfume I'd coveted for ages. I went to the perfume counter of my local department store and, with my card at the ready while the assistant was wrapping up my purchase, I decided to give myself a little spritz of my chosen scent. But instead of enjoying being bathed in a cloud of beautiful perfume, I gagged. It smelled – to me – like something from the depths of a rubbish dump. Feeling a wave of nausea, I hastily cancelled my purchase and left empty handed in search of the nearest bathroom.

Bleeding

The main advantage of the menopause is that you don't have to put up with periods any more and you can say goodbye to

PMS, forking out for sanitary products and the sheer inconvenience.

But you may be surprised – and a tad disheartened – to notice that you may still bleed from time to time during your perimenopause.

The frequency, duration and amount of bleeding varies tremendously between women during the perimenopause. In between periods, or after you thought they were long gone, you might notice some occasional spotting or brown discharge. For some, it could be as heavy as a period and last for days or even weeks.

Why does it happen?

There are many reasons why bleeding occurs. Firstly (and forgive me for stating the obvious), make sure it is definitely coming from your vagina and not your anus, as rectal bleeding has significantly different causes and treatments.

Vaginal bleeding can be triggered by a structural cause, such as fibroids or polyps, or by overgrowth of the cells lining your uterus; but for most women, vaginal bleeding is due to hormonal changes. During the perimenopause, your oestrogen levels can have greater fluctuations throughout the month and, when there are high levels of oestrogen, bleeding can sometimes occur.

For the vast majority of women, bleeding does not need to be a cause for concern. If it persists and/or you experience other symptoms – whether you are on HRT or not – then you should speak to a healthcare professional.

Brain fog

At some point, we've all walked into a room only to momentarily wonder why we were there in the first place. Brain fog describes those moments of forgetfulness, confusion or 'woolliness', where you just can't think straight. One woman recently described it to me as feeling like the shutters had come down in her brain and that she could no longer think clearly.

This can be an embarrassing symptom: I remember keeping my friend waiting for me for an hour at a coffee shop because I'd completely forgotten we were supposed to be seeing each other. I was happily pottering around the house, phone charging in another room. It was only when I went to check my emails that I saw the missed calls and messages from my friend and realised I'd forgotten. I was mortified!

But while the odd memory slip or searching around for your specs only to find you are wearing them can be funny, brain fog can also be very distressing, particularly in the workplace, where you have to appear organised. Many women worry they have dementia or even a brain tumour. Some tell me that they have forgotten to attend important meetings or have met with colleagues whose names and details they have completely forgotten, which would have never been a problem in the past.

Why does it happen?

Oestrogen and testosterone have significant roles to play in your brain. Oestrogen can increase the number of connections in your hippocampus,[6] the part of your brain important for memory and certain types of learning. Testosterone strengthens nerves in your brain and contributes to mental sharpness and clarity;[7] it also strengthens arteries that supply blood flow to your brain, which may be crucial in protecting against memory loss.

Breast tenderness

Some women experience breast tenderness, and you might find the shape of your breasts changes.

Why does it happen?

Fluctuating hormone levels are usually to blame for breast tenderness. Oestrogen can cause your breast ducts to enlarge, while progesterone causes the milk glands to swell (it is known as the pregnancy hormone, remember?), usually in tune with your menstrual cycle. A lack of oestrogen can lead to shrinkage in your breasts and your breasts might not feel as full or as round as they used to.

The bottom line is that these changes are usually harmless, but make an appointment with a healthcare professional if you notice any pain or changes that concern you. You should seek advice if pain is accompanied by a fever, you feel a hard lump that does not move, you have nipple discharge or a rash in or around your nipple, your breasts have changed shape or your skin on your breast area appears dimpled.

Breast pain? How to feel more comfortable

- **Check your bra fit.** Your bra supports your breast tissue, so it's important to make sure it fits well. Many department stores and lingerie shops offer fitting services, and if you can't make it to a shop consider a virtual fitting appointment instead.
- **Try wearing a bra in bed.** Some women find wearing a bra in bed helps to alleviate breast pain or tenderness. Sports bras are

designed to give greater support, while many brands stock sleep bras that are non-wired and softer.

- **Plan your exercise carefully.** You don't want breast tenderness to get in the way of leading an active life, so consider which exercise is best suited to you. You might find high-impact sports like running or aerobics exacerbate your symptoms, so switch to something gentle in the interim – and don't forget to look for a sports bra to support you during exercise.
- **Cut it out.** Caffeine and nicotine both stimulate breast tissue, which can make them feel more sensitive, so consider cutting down on the caffeine and cutting out nicotine altogether. In addition, too much salt in your diet can lead to water retention, which, in turn, can contribute to breast pain. Current UK guidelines are that adults should eat no more than 6g of salt a day (2.4g sodium),[8] which is around one teaspoon.
- **Hot and cold** Try heat or cold therapy – using heat packs or ice packs – to see if this brings any relief: wrapping the pack in a thin towel to help protect your skin, apply to the affected area for fifteen to twenty minutes a couple of times a day. You can alternate between hot and cold, if you find this helps.

Brittle nails
Nails can become thin or soft, meaning they can split, crack or break more easily.

Why does it happen?
Your nails are made of a protein called keratin, which gives them structure and helps keep them hard and strong. Oestrogen helps

to produce keratin so, when levels are lower, your nails may be more susceptible to breaks.

Difficulty breathing

Feeling a bit wheezy or like you can't seem to catch your breath (particularly when you are active during exercise or climbing stairs)? If you had childhood asthma, do you feel it's made a return lately?

Why does it happen?

Mucus (also known as phlegm or sputum) is part of our lungs' immune response, helping to protect us from infection by trapping irritants and allowing the body to eliminate them through coughing. Oestrogen helps with mucus production. In addition, oestrogen reduces inflammation in your lung tissues, so there can be an increase in inflammation leading to symptoms of shortness of breath or wheezing during the perimenopause and menopause.[9]

And while your lung function will naturally decline as you get older, studies have shown that there is a decrease in lung capacity after the menopause, particularly in women who had an earlier menopause.[10]

If you are experiencing shortness of breath regularly, you should see a healthcare professional to rule out other causes.

Dizziness

You may notice intermittent periods of feeling dizzy or light-headed. This can happen after bending down to put on your shoes, for example; or you may feel a bit wobbly in the shower and feel you need to steady yourself or sit down.

Why does it happen?

Oestrogen, progesterone and testosterone have an effect on the way your blood vessels widen and narrow, so, when hormone levels fluctuate, this can trigger feelings of light-headedness, pressure and dizziness. These hormones can also affect the function of your balance areas of the brain and also your inner ear.[11] To be on the safe side, however, see a healthcare professional if you've had episodes of severe dizziness, fainting or palpitations to rule out any other underlying causes.

Dry eyes

Every time you blink, your eyes release a tear film made up of water, oil and mucus that covers and lubricates your eyes. When you don't produce enough of this substance, your eyes can feel dry, with stinging, a gritty feeling (like you have something in your eye) or blurry vision. This symptom can be a real nuisance, particularly if, like me, you spend a lot of time in front of a computer screen. My own optician recently referred one of his patients to me when her eyes became so dry that she was struggling to wear her usual contact lenses.

Why does it happen?

As we get older, tear production decreases and oestrogen also plays a part in tear-film production. Research also suggests that male sex hormones (known as androgens) help to manage the delicate balance of tear production.[12]

Tips to manage dry eyes

- **Limit screen time.** When you use a laptop, tablet or smartphone you blink less, meaning your eyes can get drier. Try to take a screen break at least once an hour. But if you really can't leave your desk, close your eyes for a few minutes or blink repeatedly for a few seconds when you feel your eyes are getting dry.
- **Protect your peepers.** Cold weather and wind can cause tears to evaporate too quickly and make dry eyes worse. You could try wraparound sunglasses to protect your eyes from the elements, particularly if out running or cycling. If you are a contact-lens wearer, speak to your optician about ones that will help to keep your eyes more moist, only wear them for the recommended time and never sleep with them in. You could also keep a pair of glasses to give yourself some contact-lens-free days.
- **Know your triggers.** Do contact lenses, smoky atmospheres or pollen make your eyes itch? Keep a record of your triggers and try to avoid them where practically possible.
- **How's your humidity?** A humidifier in your home can help to keep the eyes moist, so your tears won't evaporate as quickly.
- **Look at your diet.** Omega-3 fatty acids (found in oily fish and eggs) and vitamin A (found in eggs and dairy) can both encourage healthy tear production.

Dry and itchy skin

You might find yourself noticing more wrinkles and fine lines when you look in the mirror, or that the skin all over your body feels rougher, dry and even itchy.

Why does it happen?
As oestrogen levels fall during the perimenopause and menopause, skin becomes thinner and more water is lost, leading to
more lines, a drier texture and, for some women, an itchy,
uncomfortable feeling. Chapter 6 is dedicated to dealing with
changes to skin and hair, so, if you have an itch you just can't
seem to resolve, head there for more advice.

Dry mouth, gum disease, bad breath and other oral-health symptoms

One area in which more awareness is definitely needed is the
impact of menopause on your oral health. I frequently see
women in my clinic present with oral symptoms that can be
uncomfortable, distressing and, often, embarrassing.

Why does it happen?
Oestrogen is crucial in the healthy functioning of the supporting
structures of your teeth, bones and ligaments, as well as the
mucous membranes inside your mouth.[13,14] When hormone
levels fall, this can have a direct impact on oral health, triggering
a range of issues, which include the following:

- Gingivitis (a common form of gum disease, where the gums
  become swollen, red and sore)
- Periodontitis (an infection of the gums)
- Toothache
- Dry mouth
- Burning mouth
- Tooth loss
- Halitosis (bad breath)

- An altered sense of taste, particularly for salt or sour foods
- Tooth sensitivity

EXPERT VIEW
Ways to protect your oral health during the menopause – Dr Uchenna Okoye,
Clinical Director of London Smiling Dentist Group

Dr Uchenna has worked in dentistry for more than twenty-five years and has a special expertise and interest in cosmetic dentistry. Here, she takes us through her advice on the neglected area of caring for your oral health during perimenopause and menopause.

If I asked people to name life events that can impact your oral health, I am willing to bet that menopause wouldn't feature on many lists. In fact, very few people make the link between declining hormone levels and changes inside their mouths.

But as Dr Louise has outlined, falling hormone levels can leave you at greater risk of conditions such as dryness that leaves you more vulnerable to infection, gingivitis and periodontitis.

So with this in mind, it's more important than ever to look after your oral health during the perimenopause and menopause, and here are some tips on how to do just that:

- Tackle plaque. Reducing the amount of plaque – a sticky film of bacteria that constantly forms on the tooth surface – is key to protecting your oral health during this time. If plaque is not eliminated, it can lead to problems like gingivitis and periodontitis, so it needs to be done daily at home and besides brushing, the best way to do this is to floss: you can't just rely on your dental team to do it for you during scaling and polishing.

- Think about the toothbrush you are using. Consider using rechargeable powered brushes over manual ones, as evidence suggests plaque is removed more effectively this way. Daily interdental cleaning using brushes or floss helps to control the plaque that causes gingivitis and periodontitis.

- Consider your diet. Stress, low self-esteem and fatigue during menopause mean you might be more likely to reach for a sugary treat or an alcoholic drink. But minimising sugary food and drink (wine, beer and spirits are all made from natural starch and sugar) will reduce your risk of dental decay. If you are drinking any of these, use a straw and rinse your mouth after a sugary treat.

- Don't forget to have regular check-ups. Life is busy, and it's easy for a dental check-up to drop down the list of priorities. But I can't stress enough the importance of seeing a dentist regularly for advice and treatment if needed. There is no set timing for how often this should be – frequency of visits to your dentist and hygienist should be a conversation between you and them – and don't forget to keep up a good oral-hygiene routine between visits.

- Talk to a healthcare professional about menopause treatment if you are struggling with symptoms. HRT will replace hormones and help to reduce any oral symptoms you may be experiencing. Also consider a retainer brace as early on as you can as teeth do start to shift due to collagen shrinking so this can save you money needed for more dental work later on.

Hearing issues

Tinnitus (a constant ringing or humming sound in your ears) is a really common symptom. I've seen patients who have had thoughts of self-harm and suicide because of their tinnitus, as the noise stopped them from sleeping and functioning.

Why does it happen?
There hasn't been a lot of research on the impact of menopause on tinnitus and hearing loss. However, we do know that oestrogen helps your nerves to conduct messages across neural pathways; therefore, low levels can cause your nerves to not work properly, which can lead to all sorts of symptoms, including tinnitus and hearing loss.[15]

Heart palpitations

Most people don't give their heart function a second thought, but if you notice your heart is beating more intensely than usual, or irregularly, this is a palpitation. The feeling may last for a few seconds or a couple of minutes. Palpitations can coincide with a hot flush or a night sweat (more of which in a moment), a dizzy spell, when you are feeling breathless, or they can happen on their own. Palpitations can be associated with sleep problems and also reduced quality of life.[16]

Why does it happen?
Palpitations can be due to changing or declining levels of oestrogen, which can affect the pathways in your heart through which electrical impulses travel. They can feel quite alarming, but the reassuring thing is that in most cases they are not a sign of a serious cardiac issue. However, you should see a doctor if you have any other concerns or if your palpitations:

- last for a few minutes
- are associated with shortness of breath or chest pain

- get worse over time, or start happening more often
- do not improve within three months of starting HRT.

Heartburn

Also known as acid reflux, heartburn (which, despite its name, is not a heart-related problem) is a horrible burning feeling in your chest and throat when stomach acid travels up into your oesophagus. This can leave an unpleasant taste in your mouth, give you bad breath and make you feel bloated and nauseous.

Why does it happen?

Common causes of heartburn include stress and being over-weight; however, fluctuating oestrogen levels can alter the amount of acid the stomach produces. In addition, when you are feeling stressed, the body produces more of the hormone corti-sol, which can affect your digestion. One study of 497 women found that 42 per cent of perimenopausal and 47 per cent of menopausal women suffered from heartburn.[17]

Hot flushes and night sweats

And now we come to probably the most recognisable menopause symptom: hot flushes. Let's look at what happens.

Why does it happen?

The exact cause of hot flushes isn't known, but it is thought to be related to changing oestrogen levels impacting on the areas of the brain involved in maintaining temperature.[18] Night sweats are similar to hot flushes but, as the name suggests, they only happen at night, and are accompanied by sweating.

ANATOMY OF A HOT FLUSH

1 Your brain mistakenly thinks you are overheating and starts a process to cool your body down.

2 Your temperature rises in response and blood vessels dilate to increase blood flow.

3 Your heart starts to pump out blood to the dilated vessels and you may feel heat in your core, dizziness, shortness of breath or palpitations.

4 This heat escapes from the blood vessels, with the tell-tale flush spreading to other areas of your body including your chest, neck and face.

5 You may begin to perspire to get rid of the excess heat.

6 After lasting for just a few seconds, or for several minutes, the hot flush starts to subside.

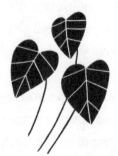

Many women have told me the only way they can cool down overnight is sleeping on the tiled bathroom floor or keeping a fan on next to their bed. Some women even carry changes of clothes with them, as they constantly sweat through what they are wearing.

Hot flushes can happen at any time – and up to several times a day. Triggers include the following:

- Spicy foods, caffeine and alcohol
- Smoking
- An existing temperature
- Stress or anxiety
- Certain cancer treatments
- Health conditions, including an overactive thyroid, diabetes and tuberculosis

Joint or muscle pains

Aches and pains in your muscles and joints are also common when going through the menopause, especially in the mornings. One patient once told me that whenever she got up in the morning, it was like walking on glass: when she walked down the stairs, every step hurt her body; at night, she got this awful, deep bone pain and felt like her bones were being wrung out.

Why does it happen?

Oestrogen works as an anti-inflammatory agent in your muscles, and it also helps to lubricate your joints.[19] So during the menopause, when oestrogen levels dip, it can cause muscle and joint pains. This is usually most common in the mornings, as this is when oestrogen levels tend to be lowest. It is likely that oestrogen has an important role in reducing incidence and severity of osteoarthritis, too.[20]

Low libido

Libido relates to your sex drive, including your level of desire and how much pleasure you get from sex and intimacy. You might find that you are just not in the mood for sex, that you feel too tired or that you have physical issues like vaginal dryness, meaning that sex has become painful.

Why does it happen?

Testosterone often is a key hormone in regulating libido, including arousal and pleasure.[21] On top of this, lower oestrogen can lead to vaginal dryness and sore, painful sex, irritability, mood changes and low self-esteem, all of which can have a knock-on effect on your sex life.

SURVEY: THE HIDDEN IMPACT OF MENOPAUSE ON RELATIONSHIPS

Barely a day goes by in my clinic without a patient telling me how menopause has stretched her relationship to breaking point.

Mood changes. Anxiety. Low libido, just like we're discussing now. Physical aches and pains. Fatigue. Low self-esteem. Any one of those symptoms can affect you; and, if you are in a relationship, they can indirectly affect the person you love as well. Sometimes, the knock-on effect of these symptoms pushes relationships beyond the point of no return, resulting in a complete and irretrievable breakdown.

I know first-hand how my symptoms tested my own marriage. And I've heard women describe how their decades-long marriages ended, while others in new relationships brimming with potential tell me how they finished before they'd ever really got started.

With the onset of perimenopause in the mid-forties, the average age of menopause at fifty-one and the peak time of divorce being between the ages of forty-five and fifty-five, it's long been assumed, but never proven, that the menopause has a clear and negative impact on divorce, separation and relationships.

So in 2022, my clinic teamed up with the Family Law Menopause Project for a landmark survey to investigate the impact of menopause on relationships. More than a thousand women who had either gone through or were currently going through a divorce took part in the poll.

Here's what we found:

- Seven in 10 women (73 per cent) blamed the menopause for the breakdown of their marriage.
- Worryingly, a further 67 per cent claimed it increased domestic abuse and arguments.
- Sadly, only a fifth of those women had sought support to talk about the perimenopause/menopause because at the time, they didn't think it was a contributing factor to the breakdown of their relationships.
- Almost 80 per cent of respondents said that their symptoms put a strain on their children and/or family life; only a third of all women had been offered treatment or HRT to relieve their symptoms despite it being the optimum treatment.
- In contrast, 65 per cent of those who were offered HRT said it had made a positive impact on their menopause-related symptoms.
- Some 70 per cent of those who had not received support or treatment said that if they had, it would have had a positive impact on their relationship and potentially avoided the breakdown of their marriage.

Of course, results like these make for concerning reading. But what I hope is that if you are having relationship difficulties right now, they will help you to open the conversation and encourage you to seek help and support.

Low mood, anxiety and depression

Psychological symptoms can be particularly difficult to deal with during perimenopause and menopause – so much so that we have a whole chapter devoted to menopause and mental health. So if this is something that is affecting you, turn to Chapter 5 for more information, tips and support.

Why does it happen?

When oestrogen falls, levels of the mood-boosting hormone serotonin fall, too, while cortisol (the primary stress hormone) rises. In addition, the effects of physical symptoms such as fatigue, hot flushes or weight gain to name a few can affect your mood and self-esteem. For example: when I found myself forgetting things at work, I used to feel completely useless: it knocked my confidence in my ability as a doctor. Then, when I got home, I would ruminate on it. The effect on my self-esteem, coupled with poor sleep because of night sweats, really affected me.

Migraines

A migraine is a moderate or severe headache, often felt as a throbbing pain and usually occurring on one side of the head. It can come with nausea or vomiting and a heightened sensitivity to light or sound, and is often debilitating, lasting anything from a few hours to a few days. Other symptoms such as slurred speech, arm or leg weakness, reduced ability to concentrate and extreme fatigue may also occur.

Migraines mainly come on without notice, but some people will have a warning sign via an 'aura' – a collective term for symptoms that occur just before the migraine comes on. These can include visual disturbances (such as seeing dark or coloured spots, flashing lights or zigzag lines), vertigo, dizziness, numbness or tingling. Some people can suffer with migraines several times a week, while others can go several years between episodes.

Why does it happen?
If you already suffer from migraines, you may have found they tended to occur just before your period (or about a week before, if you are taking the combined oral contraceptive pill).

During the perimenopause and menopause, fluctuations in your hormone levels can result in migraines occurring more frequently and being worse during the perimenopause compared to the menopause. This is because changing hormone levels (rather than the actual level) can trigger migraines.[22]

I have suffered with migraines for as long as I can remember. They were particularly bad soon after my children were born (on reflection, this is likely to have been related to the hormonal changes that occurred in my body around these times). It is always common for me to experience migraines at the weekends or on holiday, when I am relaxing more. It can be very common for migraines occur after a period of stress when you relax, although some people find that stress can trigger migraines, too. However, when I was perimenopausal, I would have horrendous migraines that lasted several days at a time. Taking a triptan (a drug used for migraines or headaches) has been the only thing that has really helped me. I also do not drink alcohol, I avoid caffeine (including chocolate), do not eat processed foods and try to go to bed and get up at the same time every day, all of which help to reduce the frequency of my migraines.

Pelvic-floor problems

If you are finding you have to cross your legs when you laugh or sneeze, in case a bit of wee comes out, or that the mere thought of jumping up and down during a workout terrifies you, then you might need to work on your pelvic floor – because you might be suffering from a condition known as stress incontinence. You might also find yourself waking several times during the night to go to the toilet (this is known as nocturia) or feel an intense urge to urinate, only for a tiny amount to come out (known as urge incontinence).

Why does it happen?

Pelvic-floor dysfunction can occur after childbirth and during the perimenopause and menopause, as oestrogen drops significantly during these times. The vagina, vulva and urinary tract are all lined with oestrogen receptor cells, and, when oestrogen is no longer in plentiful supply in the body, these areas can really suffer. As a result, the lining of your bladder and urethra (the tube that carries urine out of the body) thins and your pelvic floor – which supports your bladder, uterus (womb) and rectum – gets weaker.

You might have seen specialist sanitary products in supermarkets designed to deal with incontinence, but none of these issues should be treated as an inevitable sign of ageing, and I would always urge you to seek specialist help.

EXPERT VIEW
Pelvic-floor problems – Jane Simpson,
Pelvic-floor and Continence Nurse Specialist
and author of *The Pelvic Floor Bible*

Jane treats women and men of all ages with incontinence and pelvic-floor dysfunction. She has a special interest in areas including the menopause, stress incontinence, overactive bladder, urge incontinence, lifestyle issues to do with pelvic health, prolapse and constipation. She is one of the 'balance+ gurus' on my balance app, with regular articles and videos on all things pelvic-floor-related.

Pelvic-floor dysfunction is a global health problem: approximately 5–6 million women in the UK have experienced symptoms of the condition,[23] but, even in this day and age, it remains underreported, undertreated and taboo.

My patients tell me things like, 'I am so ashamed I wet myself'; 'I just couldn't get to the toilet in time' or, 'I don't dare to do any star jumps'; 'I have an awful dragging feeling in my vagina by the end of the day' or 'I've stopped having sex because it's so painful and dry'. Does one or even all of these statements ring a bell with you?

Childbirth and decreasing oestrogen levels at the menopause are the most common causes of pelvic floor dysfunction. We are living longer, exercising harder, having babies later and will spend about a third of our lives in post-menopause. So, it's more important than ever to love our pelvic floor!

WHAT CAN BE DONE ABOUT IT?

The most important three things to remember about pelvic floor health are: Are you using the right muscles? Are you doing your exercises regularly? Most pelvic floor problems can be cured or certainly better managed.

Pelvic-floor exercises

These are key in strengthening and maintaining pelvic-floor strength and health and should be a vital part of all our daily routines. They're also very easy to do:

- Sit on the arm of a chair or any hard surface, with your feet flat on the floor, and lean slightly forwards so that your vulval area is in contact with a firm surface.
- With your hands on your thighs, try to lift the area around your vagina and anus away from the surface you are sitting on.
- Draw up all the muscles at the same time, squeeze, lift and hold for a count of five (aim to build up to a count of ten). Let go gently and count to five, then repeat the movement again, five times.

Once a day, do ten short, sharp contractions in a rhythmic pattern of squeeze, let go, squeeze, let go, squeeze, let go.

Try to do this exercise three times a day (or at least twice) – find something that you can associate to doing the exercises: like cleaning your teeth, turning on your computer or driving to work, so you don't forget. It needs to become a habit and a normal part of your daily routine

If you think that you can't contract or relax your pelvic floor, talk to a specialist.

Seek specialist help

Where are my pelvic floor muscles and how do I find them?

A women's health physiotherapist or continence nurse specialist will be able to find out what is exactly wrong and start you on the right treatment and/or equipment, if you are struggling on your own.

Biofeedback is used in lots of different therapies to gain better awareness of muscle movements. For the pelvic floor, it is usually done using a vaginal electrode, as you contract your muscles, you get a visual response (in a clinic setting, often as a graph on the computer screen). There are now lots of things available to buy that give an element of biofeedback and help with pelvic floor strengthening. I am a fan of tools and gadgets; a bit like using your Fitbit, they can be very motivating in our busy lives. Things like vaginal weights, intravaginal devises that work with an app on your phone, small electrical stimulation devices, pants that don't involve a vaginal probe but externally stimulate the pelvic floor, and a pelvic floor educator. The most important thing is to find what works best for you.

The overactive bladder

Many people suffer with urgency or frequency of urine that sometimes ends in urge incontinence. Does the sight of your front door make you desperate for the toilet?

What can you do about it?

Pelvic floor rehabilitation alongside bladder retraining are the first steps.

The goal is to retrain the bladder by cutting the number of times you pass urine down to six to eight in a twenty-four-hour period. You can do this by following these tips.

Keep a bladder diary to see what you are drinking and make a note of how often you go to the toilet. Drinking too much tea, coffee, alcohol and fizzy drinks may make things worse. Try to steadily lengthen the time between your visits to the toilet.

Drink about 1.5 litres of fluid per day – a bit more if you are exercising. If this isn't working, seek help from a healthcare professional, as you may need further investigations such as a urine test and/or medication.

Vaginal Prolapse

About thirty to fifty per cent of women over fifty have a degree of prolapse. This can be helped by pelvic floor rehabilitation, avoiding constipation, trying not to be overweight and avoiding very heavy lifting. While you are improving your pelvic floor strength a vaginal pessary can be very helpful; they are inserted into the vagina to support your prolapse, initial fitting is best done by a healthcare professional, but disposable ones can be bought online. Pessaries can be worn all the time or just for sport, I always say you wouldn't go for a run without your sports bra, so why not look after your vagina the same way? Ultimately and always the last resort is surgery.

Urinary-tract infections

Our urinary-tract system is responsible for removing waste products from our bodies via urine. A urinary-tract infection (UTI) refers to an infection in any part of this system, including your ureters (tubes that carry urine from your kidneys to your bladder), bladder and urethra.

A UTI can be very uncomfortable, leading to a burning sensation, pain when urinating, smelly or cloudy urine and lower abdominal and/or back pain.

Why does it happen?

Your body's protection from bugs that infiltrate the vaginal and urinary areas gets weaker due to reduced oestrogen levels. UTIs happen when harmful bacteria spread to these areas and overwhelm the natural defences of more helpful ones. It is known that oestrogen deficiency (occurring in the menopause) can contribute to urinary symptoms and also increase your risk of recurrent UTIs.[24] Oestrogen has been shown to stimulate secretion of anti-microbial substances in your bladder and vaginal cells, which then improve immunity and reduce the risk of infections.[25] We are currently doing some exciting research in this area with consultant urological surgeon Prof Chris Harding.

It can be common to experience symptoms of a UTI even if you have no actual infection, due to the lack of oestrogen in your bladder and surrounding tissues.

CASE STUDY: USING HER EXPERIENCE
TO SUPPORT WOMEN THROUGH THE
MENOPAUSE – ROWAN'S STORY

Rowan was a successful businesswoman who loved the outdoors. When she started to experience a raft of physical and psychological symptoms that affected her confidence and her career, she was put through a multitude of tests – but no one even mentioned perimenopause or menopause. Having finally got the help she needed following a referral to a specialist clinic, Rowan now volunteers at a menopause support group.

'I lost my father when I was thirty-nine. He had brought me up, and I had cared for him before he died, and it hit me particularly hard. So when I had the symptoms of what I now know as perimenopause, I initially thought it was grief. But then it went on, and on – even two years later I'd have emotional days when I couldn't stop crying.

'I had been a fit and active outdoor person my whole life and had been working in the equine industry, running a busy event yard, teaching and riding semi-professionally. Yet here I was in my early forties, suffering from broken sleep, anxiety and lost confidence. It began to have a serious impact on my riding career, as the anxiety became unbearable and I had panic attacks. I felt so unwell all the time – like someone had knocked me off my feet.

'The only thing I knew – or thought I knew – about the menopause at that point was that I wouldn't have to worry about it until I was well into my fifties, and then it would just involve getting a bit hot and sweaty. How hard could that be? I spent half my life sweating doing physical work, anyway. I had no idea it could hit women of my age, or even in their twenties.

'I'm sure now that by the time I was forty-two I was perimeno-pausal. Hot flushes weren't a big thing for me, but I was running a temperature and felt overheated the whole time. I developed urinary-tract infections – I got electric shock pains through my pelvic area, had a really painful pelvis with cramping. I thought I was diabetic because I was really thirsty and wanted to go to the loo all the time.

'I went to see a GP because I thought I was run down. It was having a real impact on my life. I'd stopped competitive riding, but I was still trying to work and be active and do my day job. I had night sweats; I'd be shivering; I'd be woken up with heart palpitations, which was really unnerving.

'The GP ordered blood tests and everything came back negative. Further down the line, I was tested for Lyme disease, connective-tissue disorders, Addison's disease – but nobody even mentioned menopause or perimenopause.

'I said to the doctor that I thought it was my hormones – that I thought my oestrogen and testosterone were low – and asked if I could be tested for that. He couldn't even look at me. He turned away and said I'd have to talk to someone who knew something about that.

'At this stage I was really struggling. This wasn't like a cold or flu, something that would go away in a few weeks. It was constant.

'I saw another GP and she gave me HRT. But I wasn't given any information about it. She asked me if I wanted patches, gel or tablets. How was I supposed to know? I said I'd try tablets, so she wrote the prescription and off I went.

'Within three or four days, my temperature had come down, my dizziness and nausea had gone and I thought, "Thank God, it's worked". But after several months, the symptoms came back again

– and my muscles ached, brain fog crept in and I felt utterly exhausted all the time. I went back to the GP. I had done some research and now knew I needed body-identical HRT – and a much higher dose.

'My life changed when I watched a menopause documentary and found a menopause specialist. I had to wait three months for the appointment and by that time I had been diagnosed with chronic fatigue. I tried to carry on, and then I slipped a disc in my back. I couldn't work – I couldn't stay awake; I was at rock bottom.

'When I got to the specialist menopause clinic, I finally felt listened to. They understood what was going on, and the help I needed. I was told to keep increasing the dose of the oestrogen every two weeks until I felt better. I was on testosterone as well, and, after several months, I felt great. All my symptoms had eased, the chronic fatigue had lifted, the brain fog had gone and I was back to teaching. It took longer to sort out the progestogen, but I feel brilliant.

'Now I volunteer at my local GP practice running menopause-support meetings. This isn't just a meet-up-and-have-coffee thing – it's a place where women can come and gain more knowledge about the menopause and how to deal with their symptoms with up-to-date medical information. I've also set up a Facebook group.

'I'm very lucky to feel as good as I do now, but it hasn't been without a fight. Women shouldn't have to go through this. We've got to come out of the dark ages, and there's still a long way to go.'

Genitourinary syndrome of the menopause (GSM) and vaginal dryness

This is where the tissue lining your vagina thins and becomes drier. Symptoms include soreness, redness, irritation and inflammation or pain during sex. But it's not just an issue if you are sexually active; you might also feel pain or discomfort when using a tampon, riding a bike, sitting down or even when wearing trousers or underwear. Other symptoms include vaginal discharge and itching.

It is estimated that around two thirds of menopausal women will experience vulvovaginal atrophy, which is a change in vaginal and vulval tissues due to menopause-associated oestrogen reduction.[26] We tend to use the term genitourinary syndrome of the menopause (GSM), however, as vulvovaginal atrophy refers to only vaginal and vulval changes, whereas GSM covers vaginal and vulval changes, plus associated problems like urinary-tract symptoms, which are also very common.[27]

Why does it happen?
Oestrogen is a natural lubricant, so falling levels can leave the tissues around your vulva and vagina more dry and less flexible. Symptoms can present in the earlier years of your perimenopause or may not occur at all until years after your menopause. While we spend a lot of time focusing on symptoms like hot flushes, vaginal dryness can be one of those hidden issues. Women often don't want to talk about it, or don't know its links to the menopause. But it's so important we do talk about it; symptoms usually persist forever without treatment, after the end of the menopause, but it is a symptom we can and do successfully treat (see p. 213 for more on this).

3

Menopause and Family History

Four things you will learn in this chapter:

1. Can you predict when you might become menopausal –
   and does family history have anything to do with it?

2. The factors that won't influence your menopause

3. How to talk about the menopause with older members
   of your family

4. If you have children, how to have constructive
   conversations with them

My mother, Ann, is an absolute life force.

Even at her age, she is still working as a LAMDA (London Academy
of Music and Dramatic Art) examiner and shows no sign of slowing
down as she gets older (or as she matures, as she prefers to say).

Drama and performance have been her life's passion, ever
since she first set foot on stage at the tender age of five. She

studied speech and drama at the prestigious Royal Academy of Music and, after numerous theatre roles, she later moved into drama teaching.

It was when my mother was in her forties and teaching drama in London that she started to experience terrible fatigue. Nothing out of the ordinary for a working mother with three young children, you may say, but it got to the point where even getting out of bed and getting dressed in the morning felt like the most enormous effort.

My mother is an incredibly strong person; she had to be. Widowed at a young age, she was the main breadwinner when many of her peers stayed at home and were not working. It must have been very frightening for her experiencing these symptoms without someone to share the burden, and knowing she had to keep things together for the sake of her family.

She didn't actually realise it was the menopause at first, chiefly because she didn't have any hot flushes or night sweats. While she didn't recall much of her own mother's menopause, one memory that stuck in her head was of a family friend who suffered from hot flushes, the sweat pouring down her face. These were down to menopause but, because my mum didn't experience the same all those years later, she didn't realise that she too was menopausal.

Mum went to see her doctor, who told her, on account of her age, that she was going through the 'change', as it was so often referred to back then. 'You'll get through it,' he said, and sent her on her way.

'One didn't talk about women's medical issues in those days,' Mum recalls. 'When I was little, we didn't even call them periods; we would call them "the curse", and practically whisper it.

As I got older, people would talk about the "change", but I didn't really know what the word menopause meant.'

But Mum still didn't feel any better, so she did what I often advise women to do – she saw another doctor for a second opinion. This time, the doctor suggested she tried taking HRT. She didn't even know what HRT stood for at that point but was so desperate for her old life back that she was willing to try anything.

And Mum is still taking HRT to this day, thanks to her foresight in going back to ask for help, and that forward-thinking second doctor. Many different GPs have tried to stop her taking it over the years, but she has always pushed back and continued with it.

Unfortunately, many women through the decades were not so fortunate as her.

One of the criticisms I've got used to being levelled at me is why am I making such a racket about the menopause? Women have gone through it for thousands of years and have got on with it – and so should we. And not everyone suffers with menopause symptoms, so why do we suddenly all need to talk about it? Mine is a private clinic, after all, so many people think it must make good business sense that women are encouraged to seek help.

But that completely misses the point.

I only started my own clinic because I couldn't achieve what I wanted to do within the NHS. And before I started that, I set up my own website (then called menopausedoctor.co.uk), where women could get access to information for free.

It never was, is or will be about money for me.

What I want is for you, for me, for everyone, wherever they live to feel *able* to talk about it if they want to, and not to feel like this is something to bear alone if symptoms are difficult.

In 1931, life expectancy at birth was 61.8 years for females in England and Wales[28] (it now stands at 90.2 years for females born in 2022[29]). After the Second World War, however, our general health and life expectancy improved, so women were more likely to live long enough to go through the menopause. But while our health got better in those post-war years, our willingness to talk about it – particularly women's health issues – still lagged behind. A lot of suffering must have been going on behind closed doors after the children went to school and husbands were at work in the days when a woman was generally expected to stay at home.

But even in the 1980s, when my mum was going through her menopause, it wasn't getting talked about. She says that when she's spoken to women of her generation in recent years about the menopause, often the first thing they say is that they got through it fine with no symptoms. But then, on reflection, they will remember the brain fog, the tiredness or the anxiety. Many of her friends who do not take HRT are currently struggling with poor sleep, joint pains and urinary symptoms, and some have recently been diagnosed with dementia.

I was in my early teens when my mum was menopausal, and I remember her being quite tired, irritable and argumentative – but I was also hormonal, so thought many of her outbursts were due to the way I was behaving rather than the way she was feeling. However, I don't ever remember discussing the menopause, or any other women's health issues around that time, with my mum.

We've done a 360 since then – I often talk to my mum about my work and menopause in general, and she's even appeared on my podcast (see Resources, p. 357). She is a great advocate for

HRT and I am sure that it has enabled her to live a really reward-ing, energetic and stimulating life.

Talking to female family members about menopause in general is so important. And that's why I wanted this chapter to have a three-generation perspective – my mum's, my own and my oldest daughter's (Jess).

We'll be looking at genetic influences on your menopause, dispelling some common myths about other factors that can determine when you start your menopause and looking at ways to start the conversation – and keep it going.

Is it possible to predict when you'll become menopausal?

There's no simple answer when it comes to the menopause.

We know the average age for menopause onset in the UK is fifty-one, but it is exactly that – an average; and of the thousands of women we see at my clinic every year, a large number are in their forties, thirties and even younger. My youngest patient was twelve when she became menopausal. This is extremely rare, but her ovaries had not developed properly, so did not function. Another patient was only fifteen when she was diagnosed with a rare type of cancer in her thigh. The radiotherapy and chemo-therapy she received as part of her cancer treatment resulted in her ovaries no longer functioning, so she became menopausal as a teenager. No woman is too young to become menopausal.

So how will you know when the menopause will happen for you?

....

Certain treatments due to cancer or another health condition may lead to an earlier menopause than you were expecting (if this is you, please head to Chapters 7 and 8 for some tailored information and advice).

But sometimes your genes can give a good indication of when you may go through a 'natural' menopause. And that is why you might find during an initial consultation that you are asked when your mother, grandmother and other female family members went through theirs.

If there's a pattern of earlier menopause in close family members, we often find in clinic that subsequent generations follow suit. This family link has been explored in research over the decades: in 1995, a study looked at the likelihood of an early menopause in women with and without a family history of early menopause (defined as younger than forty-six for the purposes of the study).[30] Overall, 129 (37.5 per cent) of the early-menopause cases reported a family history of menopause before age forty-six years in a mother, sister, aunt or grandmother. Risk for early menopause associated with family history was greatest for those who had a sister who'd had an earlier menopause.

Genetics is only one part of determining age of menopause, though, so asking your relatives about their menopause is just a guide.[31]

Some factors that *won't* influence when you start your menopause

The age you started your periods

Periods usually begin around the age of twelve, compared to sixteen-and-a-half in the 1860s.[32] While global studies suggest that girls are starting at an earlier age these days, there is a lack of consensus as to whether there is a link between when you start your periods and when you reach the menopause.

Taking the contraceptive pill or using the Mirena coil

Birth control contains synthetic forms of oestrogen and/or progesterone: the combined contraceptive pill contains both, while the progesterone-only pill and the Mirena coil contain a type of progesterone. While using the contraceptive pill or Mirena coil won't influence when you start the menopause, one thing to bear in mind is that contraception can sometimes mask menopausal symptoms. Also, many lead to periods changing or even stopping, so that it can be really difficult to determine when you are menopausal or perimenopausal.

Taking HRT

Some women think that taking HRT during perimenopause delays the start of menopause. This is not the case. If your symptoms return when you stop taking HRT, it is not because you have been taking hormones, but because you would still be having symptoms of the menopause at that time, even if you had never taken it.

Talking to your mother or other female relatives about the menopause

Timeout #1: Questions to ask female family members

- When did they become menopausal?
- What sort of symptoms did they experience?
- Can they remember when other female family members became menopausal, such as their own mother, grandmother, sister or aunt?

Maybe you already have the kind of relationship with your mother or other female family members where no topic is off-limits. In that case, you've probably had the menopause talk, which is fantastic. But so many families hit a verbal roadblock when it comes to talking about so-called 'women's issues' between the generations.

I liken it to pregnancy: before your baby arrives, well-meaning friends and family focus on the positives as you prepare for a life-changing event. It's usually only after the birth that the floodgates open – stories of difficult labour, of colic and crying through the night, the overwhelming tiredness. Stories come tumbling out, as though you have been given membership to a secret society.

But why do we have to wait until after the event to talk about these issues when a frank chat with female family members can help to prepare for our own perimenopause and menopause? Finding out about their menopause history can often (although not always) give you an indication of when you can expect to go through your own menopause.

Perhaps, however, your mother or grandmother are not forthcoming when it comes to their health and wellbeing, in which case the following tips will help you to tread carefully and find out the information you need.

Easy does it

Think about *when* you want to have the conversation. The next family reunion where there are lots of grandchildren and long-lost cousins may not be an opportune time to speak to your mother or grandmother about their health. Find a quiet moment on your next visit, or pop round for a coffee. If you can, do it face to face, so you can pick up on any verbal cues.

Ask open-ended questions

I always try to ask open-ended questions during consultations because it is important my patients feel comfortable and know they are entering into a two-way conversation. And the same goes for any time you broach a sensitive subject with a loved one. If you rely on closed questions, they usually elicit a yes/no answer only, and you won't find out as much information. Who-, what-, where-, when- and why-type questions are a good place to start, such as 'How would you describe your menopause?' 'About how old were you?' 'What sort of symptoms did you have?' 'What sticks out in your mind about that time?'

If they have a lot to say, ask if you can record it . . .

When you are concentrating intently on what the other person is saying, or furiously writing notes, it is easy to miss important points, and it can also interrupt the flow of a conversation. Hitting record on your phone means you can listen back to the conversation later, fully absorb it and check there's nothing you missed.

. . . and keep a note of the answers for future generations

You may not have any symptoms to suggest you are perimenopausal yet, so jot down the answers and keep them for when you need them. And if you or female siblings have your own children, keep a copy for them, too, so you have as complete a family picture as possible.

EXPERT VIEW
Talking to your family about the menopause – Julia Samuel,
Psychotherapist and author

When I was sketching ideas for this chapter, I knew I wanted to bring in my own family's multi-generational experience of menopause. It was important to me that the chapter was written from my perspective as a doctor, as a menopausal woman, as a mother and as a daughter. But I also wanted it to include some expert advice in navigating those difficult conversations within family units. And who better to provide this insight than Julia Samuel, eminent psychotherapist and founder patron of the charity Child Bereavement UK.

Julia and I first met in 2022, a few months before she appeared as a guest on my podcast; I honestly could have talked to her all day. Her expertise, wisdom and compassion truly mark her out as a leader in her field, and I'm delighted to share her contribution to this book:

Families are constantly going through change, such as starting school, moving house, changing jobs or new relationships. But it is at peak points of change that they struggle – because it puts pressure not just on the individual member going through that change, but on the whole family system.

Mid-life and menopause tends to be one of those peak points of change for women. If you have children, they may be teenagers and acting out, you may have older parents or relatives who rely on you or you may be coping with the feelings of someone who is very much a sexual being, but who may be feeling invisible.

Why you need to be open and honest

In all families, across the generations and sexes, we need to have conversations and share information about periods, about sexual health and menopause.

Close, loving family relationships are based on trust, and that trust is built on honesty. The absolute key for all families is to have open and honest communication, and the same is true when it comes to your menopause.

When we try to 'protect' or shield our children or loved ones by not telling them the truth, either because we don't think they need to or that they should know, that leads to questions.

Why is Mum in a bad mood? Why is she slamming doors?

If we aren't being honest, their imaginations will fill in the gaps, rather than knowing the truth – that Mum is going through a hard time because she is menopausal.

Don't be tempted to hide your symptoms away, as that can lead children or other family members to start believing these changes could somehow be their fault.

How to broach the menopause with children

How you share information with your children or younger family members is key to their understanding. The main thing is to use straightforward language – now is not the time for complicated metaphors.

It could be something as simple as: 'When women like me normally get to their forties and fifties, we go through hormonal changes. That means we are no longer fertile, and the hormonal changes mean we can be more short-tempered than usual, have great surges of energy or no energy at all.'

Signpost potential symptoms and, if you have any, talk about them in straightforward terms.

Don't forget to create your own coping mechanisms

When we think about 'coping', often it is about wanting to have control.

Yet perhaps the most difficult aspect of the menopause is the sheer unpredictability of it.

We might have an idea of when the menopause might happen, but we don't know exactly when. We don't know what type of symptoms we can expect, and, if we do have symptoms, they can happen at any time.

You might feel a sense of rising panic at the thought of a work meeting because you might have a hot flush or forget what you were going to say; or the thought of going to a family event fills you with dread because you feel irritable.

When this happens, you need to delve into your own toolbox of coping mechanisms that are less about finding complete control, and more about finding a sense of calm. This toolbox could contain things such as simple breathing exercises, or it could be connecting with others. The important thing is to find something that works for you.

SURVEY: WHY WE NEED TO TALK ABOUT THE MENOPAUSE MORE AT HOME

When I was putting my survey together, one of the key areas I knew it had to cover was the menopause conversations that happen (or don't happen) in the home.

The findings confirmed my suspicions: 75 per cent of respondents said the menopause was never discussed in their home when they were growing up.

5 per cent recalled it being discussed once, 19 per cent said it was discussed occasionally, but just 1 per cent said it was discussed on a regular basis.

The survey also drilled down into specific family relationships, and the results were pretty mixed.

A third said they have/had never discussed the menopause with their mother, just over a third (38 per cent) said they had occasionally, 13 per cent had once, and 12 per cent had never discussed it at all.

The lack of discussion seemed to widen among the generations, with 83 per cent of respondents saying they had never discussed the menopause with a grandmother.

Lack of knowledge and feelings of shame

When asked what the key barriers (if any) to family menopause discussions were, a lack of knowledge was the most common reason, followed by embarrassment, lack of communication, being short on time and feelings of shame around the topic.

Among the comments were some really encouraging stories about women who are making a concerted decision to be more open about their experiences.

'My late mother never discussed the menopause,' one respondent recalled.

'She was widowed at 48 and stoically managed to raise her family, she probably put anything amiss down to grief. I do wish we had had conversations about menopause – I make sure that my children are aware of the symptoms.'

'My mum lost her own mother very early and didn't see her experience menopause. Mum then had an awful menopause experience herself, which was never discussed with her friends. It made my sisters and I much more aware of our own symptoms when they began and we often discuss our symptoms, feelings and experiences with each other.'

'I talk about the menopause with my friends constantly but I must talk more with my two sons,' another respondent admitted.

The importance of menopause education

I couldn't agree more that younger people must be part of the conversation, not just in the home, but the classroom as well.

After a lot of campaigning, in 2020, menopause was added to the Relationship and Sex Education curriculum in secondary schools in England.[33]

It's a great start, but these lessons are too valuable to be just a tick-box exercise.

So if you have teenage children of your own who are participating in these lessons, check in with them. How are they going? What areas are they covering? If you have a parent–teacher meeting coming up, make a point of discussing it then as well.

And if you are reading this and are part of our incredible teaching profession, ask yourself: what *do* we teach about the menopause in my school? Could we be doing more?

CASE STUDY: BROACHING MENOPAUSE WITH YOUR FAMILY – EMMA'S STORY

Emma started having perimenopausal symptoms at thirty-six. But, like many of us, she didn't really discuss menopause much growing up. Here, she tells how she is looking to change the narrative with her own children.

'Growing up, menopause really wasn't a topic of conversation. I vaguely remember my mum realising that she hadn't had a period for a while, and that was about it as far as the menopause chat went.

'When my perimenopause started, I wasn't prepared. If I'm honest, I didn't really know what the word "perimenopause" actually meant until it happened to me, and I don't think I was that unusual, as where was the mention of menopause at school?

'I didn't know at the time that earlier menopause can run in families: it turned out that while my mum went through the menopause in her forties and fifties, my grandmother had an early menopause like me. I never knew that until I was experiencing symptoms myself.

'There have been tough times but, overall, I see menopause as a second spring, an opportunity to reassess and evaluate and move forwards feeling more empowered, with a strong sense of self-awareness of who I am as a woman.

'Experiencing the menopause this early, before any of my friends, was quite an isolated place, but I now try to do something positive. I can be a source of support for my friends and be open, so they will never feel alone. I often get calls and messages because people know they can ask me anything.

'One aspect I was determined to change was around educating my children about the menopause. I have four sons and I've spoken to them all about what happens and what I have gone through. They ask how I am and if I need any help. They have been so respectful and I'm so proud of that. While they won't experience the menopause themselves, they will grow up with a working knowledge, and I think that is so important.'

Talking to teens about menopause

Talking about menopause isn't just for older generations. If we want to change the narrative around menopause, that starts in the classroom.

As a menopause specialist and the mother of three daughters, you'd think I'd be a pro at talking all things menopause with my family – but, while we *do* talk about it a lot, there is always room for improvement.

It is so important that younger members of society know about menopause, so we can normalise it. As Emma (the case study above) says – just because her four sons won't go through it themselves, that doesn't mean they don't need to know about it.

Another reason for talking to younger people about menopause is, if you have children and are menopausal, they may have picked up on changes in you and be wondering what is happening.

Here is some advice on how to broach the subject.

Pick your moment

I find my daughters are so exhausted at the end of the school day that they just want to collapse in front of the TV and are too distracted to talk. The pace can be slower at weekends, so I often find that is a good time for catch-up-type conversations. Alternatively, invite your teens out for a walk and a talk, or, if you have a car journey together ahead of you, that can be a good time for a chat.

Mind your language

Often, it is difficult to relate physical and psychological symptoms when the other person isn't going through it, so you need to think about the language you use to describe them.

When I've had a particularly bad migraine in the past, well-meaning friends assume it is the type of headache that simply goes away after taking a couple of paracetamols. Those of you reading this who also suffer from migraines know that really isn't the case, and so it is easy to feel annoyed or unheard. But look at it this way: if you've never had a migraine in your life, how would you know how it feels? The natural thing to do is to relate it to your own experience, which could be the odd tension-type headache that can be helped with some over-the-counter painkillers.

So when it comes to explaining menopause symptoms, get descriptive. Rather than simply stating 'I have fatigue', try, 'I feel like I have jet lag most mornings'; or if you have hot flushes, take the other person through exactly how it makes you feel when you have one: 'I feel like I've done a half-hour workout in thirty seconds' or, 'You know the feeling of heat hitting you when you step off a plane in a hot country? That's how intense a hot flush can be for me.' This way, you are building a picture for them of something they can, perhaps, identify with.

Find common ground

Don't forget that puberty is a time of huge upheaval: bodily changes, mood changes, new feelings that can be confusing. Sounds a bit like menopause, doesn't it? Leverage the fact that you are both going through times of hormonal change to make it relatable.

Think about how to support each other

If you have teenagers, it can feel like you spend most mornings trying to coax them out of bed. But cut them some slack – during adolescence, we secrete melatonin (the chemical that helps to regulate our circadian rhythm) later at night than in earlier childhood, which can leave teenagers sleepier in the morning. And you might be struggling with getting going in the mornings, too, thanks to fatigue or night sweats. Think of ways that you can help each other. It might be that you give yourself a fifteen-minute window to get things ready the night before (like breakfast items, making a packed lunch, leaving uniforms and work clothes laid out ready to go). Being more organised will make it less likely that tempers will fray and give you more time to talk.

And remember to prioritise yourself. If you are struggling with symptoms, ensure you see a healthcare professional who can give you the advice and treatment that is right for you. Many of us put our own health on the back burner and prioritise our family's. However, it is crucial that we are as fit and as healthy as possible, so we can help and support our family optimally. So if you are experiencing perimenopausal or menopausal symptoms, make sure you receive help.

Any questions?

Leave gaps in the conversation to allow for questions, and end by letting your child (or children) know they can ask follow-up questions at any time.

CASE STUDY: MENOPAUSE FROM A
TEEN PERSPECTIVE – JESS'S STORY

I'm giving the last word to my daughter Jess, to give you a sense of menopause through her eyes. Her story lays bare how difficult it can be for younger family members and, as she explains, how talking openly about menopause has really helped our family unit.

'I can clearly remember when I first noticed changes in Mum's behaviour. It was absolutely horrible. I was about thirteen at the time and remember thinking that my parents were going to have to break up because my mum was just so irrational and argumentative. I used to worry about what it would be like if I went to live with her if they did get divorced.

'The atmosphere could be so uncomfortable. I remember her having an argument with my dad when we were on a family holiday to London: Dad hadn't done anything wrong, but Mum was venting to me afterwards about how awful he was. But it literally sounded like some nonsense babble; I couldn't make sense of anything she was saying at all.

'Pretty soon after came that evening when my sister asked Mum outright if she was on her period because she was so grumpy. That must have been a moment of realisation for Mum because after she started taking HRT, she was a completely different person: it was amazing and made me realise how irrational she had been. Any "issues" in my parents' relationship completely went away. It was all because she was menopausal.

'Ever since, and as you would expect because of Mum's job, we do talk about menopause and women's health as a family. I have a lovely relationship with my family, and we are all very open, and I think it's so important to talk about things like that. Both of my grandmas have benefited so much from taking HRT, and we often talk about how they're walking adverts for it!

'Talking about menopause as a family has been so important because I've never been taught about the menopause formally in an educational setting, other than being told, "It's when your periods stop", which is awful.

'I don't just talk about the menopause with my family: I talk a lot with my friends, too. For me, it's just another standard topic of conversation, which is definitely due to my mum. I think that attitude has helped a lot of my friends as well: I talk about it with no shame and that's helped them to learn more and see there is no taboo surrounding the menopause. However, I know it can be hard for some of them to get their own parents and grandparents to talk freely about the menopause, even though it affects everyone, directly or indirectly. I know lots of women seem to think menopause is something they shouldn't talk about – that it is a personal thing, that they don't want/need any help and that they "can manage it by themselves".

'If you've picked up this book because you want to know how to talk to your children, nieces, nephews or even your own parents about the menopause, my advice would be that the more you talk about it, the more you normalise it. I was only thirteen, but I'd already realised that Mum was acting differently, so talking about things will help. I think it's really important to speak freely about it to remove any stigma or taboo for your children or family. Menopause isn't some massive elephant in the room. The language you use can be important, too; when I talk to my friends about it, I talk about it being a long-term hormone deficiency.

'And I know from my mum that it isn't just about talking to family and friends, but talking to professionals, too, about getting some help. You might buy a fan for your hot flushes, but this can be like putting a plaster over the problem. When you get the right help and get the correct treatment, then those symptoms will no longer be an issue at all, so things like your fan will be redundant!'

4

HRT: Everything You Need to Know

Four things you will learn in this chapter:

1. The facts: what HRT is, and the benefits it can bring, from protecting our hearts to helping our bones; plus, emerging research on dementia

2. Exclusive research: we take a closer look at public perceptions of HRT and access to it

3. Setting the record straight on any risks of HRT

4. Practical advice – how and when to take HRT, tackling temporary side effects and expert advice on everything, including breastfeeding while taking HRT and whether it is ever too late to start taking it

Without taking HRT, my life would look very different indeed.

If I had still been fatigued, brain-fogged, ill-tempered and plagued by migraines, I wouldn't have had the energy or the confidence to start my own menopause clinic, or establish a charity, a non-profit research society and the Newson Health Menopause Society, a society for healthcare professionals. I wouldn't have had the energy to raise three daughters. And I know for a fact I wouldn't have had the mental clarity and focus to sit down and write this book.

Before I started taking HRT, it was like I had a voice in my head giving me permission to be short-tempered. Fatigue and brain fog were due to the pressures of work, I thought. Then, once I realised I was perimenopausal, I did my research, weighed up my benefits and risks and decided HRT was the right option for me.

But when I went to my local GP he told me (incorrectly) that he couldn't prescribe HRT for me, because it was 'dangerous'. He was worried about the perceived breast cancer risk and was not prepared to discuss with me the many benefits of taking HRT. Instead, he offered me antidepressants to help with my low mood.

Antidepressants were the last thing I needed, so I had to seek help elsewhere. I found a private doctor who is a menopause specialist. He listened to me and gave me the prescription of HRT that I both wanted and needed.

That was back in 2017, and I've been taking HRT ever since. It's no exaggeration to say it has been the most important decision I've ever made in regard to my future health and wellbeing.

You may well be reading this knowing you're perimenopausal or menopausal and feeling fed up with the toll it's taking on your body, mind, work and relationships. Maybe you are unsure of how HRT works and if it is suitable for you. Or you are already taking HRT and want more information about it. And after years of misinformation, you might also have some important questions about how safe and effective it is.

This is the chapter where you will find the answers.

What is HRT?

HRT stands for hormone replacement therapy. Currently only available on prescription in the UK, HRT comes in dozens of different types of doses and methods – because the type of hormones you need and the doses you are given vary from person to person.

All types of HRT will contain oestrogen. If you still have a uterus, you will need to take progesterone (known as micronised progesterone or a synthetic progestogen) with the oestrogen, as taking oestrogen on its own can thicken the lining of your womb and increase the risk of uterine cancer. Some women may also benefit from testosterone.

HRT containing oestrogen alone is known, not surprisingly, as oestrogen-only HRT. HRT containing both oestrogen and progesterone is known as combined HRT.

Replacement oestrogen can be given in various ways – either as a skin patch (which looks a bit like a plaster), as a gel or spray or as a tablet that you swallow. Patches, gels and sprays are known as transdermal HRT, which means that they bypass the liver and are absorbed directly into the bloodstream. This means there is no risk of blood clot and this method has fewer side effects. Oral oestrogen needs to be digested and metabolised, so it works differently from that given through the skin. It is also easier to alter the dose of oestrogen when it is given as a patch, gel or spray, compared to a tablet.

The type of oestrogen I usually prescribe is 17 beta-oestradiol, which has the same molecular structure as the oestrogen produced in your body by your ovaries; it is termed 'body identical'. This is the most natural type of HRT to use.

The safest type of replacement progesterone is micronised progesterone; this is body identical (branded as Utrogestan in the UK) and it comes in a capsule that you swallow (occasionally, this progesterone can also be used vaginally, but it is not licensed to be used in this way). An alternative way to receive a progestogen is to have the Mirena coil inserted into your uterus. This is also a very effective contraceptive, and it needs replacing after five years.

Another option is an oral tablet that contains body-identical oestrogen and micronised progesterone and is branded as Bijuve in the UK.

If you are experiencing low sex drive and HRT alone is not helping, testosterone can often be beneficial (in addition to the oestrogen).[34] And in my clinical experience, testosterone can also help with other symptoms, such as fatigue, brain fog and low energy. It is available in a gel, cream or implant, and, while it is not currently licensed as a treatment for women in the UK, many NHS and private healthcare professionals prescribe it 'off-license'. This means that there is not a license for its use but this does not mean it is unsafe. We often prescribe medications "off-license", for example, medications to children and many migraine medications.

Benefits of HRT

HRT has two key benefits.

Firstly, by replacing the missing hormones and correcting the hormone deficiency, it eases physical and psychological symptoms. In my case, it took a few months and some adjustments of dosage before I started to feel like myself again.

Secondly – and this is a major benefit that we all need to talk about more – HRT helps to protect your long-term health. The bulk of scientific evidence – from preclinical, clinical and epidemiologic studies and also randomised clinical trials – clearly indicates that individualised HRT is usually useful and rarely dangerous. Following simple and well-established rules, usually involving prescribing body-identical hormones, HRT benefits outweigh all the possible risks.[35]

HRT replaces the missing hormones when you are menopausal. And when hormone levels fluctuate during the perimenopause, HRT is about topping them up. Having adequate oestradiol works to improve the function of your body, as the HRT tops up the missing oestradiol in your body.

The accelerated ageing that occurs with low oestradiol levels increases future risk of disease. This is related to the increased inflammation that occurs as low oestradiol stimulates the immune cells to work less efficiently. The low-grade inflammation that occurs increases the risk of inflammatory diseases – these include cardiovascular disease, osteoporosis, Alzheimer's disease, clinical depression and even some types of cancer. Parkinson's has also been shown to increase in women who have an early menopause.

HRT and osteoporosis

Bone tissue is made up of cells and blood vessels that help the bone grow and repair itself. The amount of bone tissue you have is known as bone density and is a measure of how strong and healthy your bones are. By your late thirties, your bone density starts to naturally decrease. This loss can make your bones weaker, less pliable and therefore more susceptible to breaking.

An estimated 3 million people in the UK have osteoporosis – a condition that weakens the bones and makes them more likely to break. Yet alarmingly, osteoporosis is often referred to as a 'silent disease', as so few people are aware that they have it until they suffer a fracture.

The risk factors for osteoporosis are numerous, but sex and age are key. An estimated one in two women (who do not take HRT) over fifty *worldwide* will develop osteoporosis, compared to one in five men. One in three post-menopausal women (not taking HRT) will sustain an osteoporotic fracture. And this is also where the menopause comes into play, because women are more affected by a loss of bone strength in the years during the perimenopause and after the menopause, as oestrogen (the key hormone for protecting and maintaining bone density) rapidly declines during this time. Bone is then breaking down at a faster rate than the body can grow new bone tissue.

In addition to sex and age, a family history of osteoporosis means you are more susceptible to this condition, but there are other factors that will increase your chance of having osteoporosis, too. Habits such as smoking and heavy drinking can damage the bone-building cells, while a diet lacking the important nutrients calcium and vitamin D does not give the body what it needs to grow new bone tissue.

Correcting the hormone deficiency via HRT helps to protect the bones from weakening due to lack of oestrogen and can reduce the risk of fragility fractures.[36,37]

HRT is, in fact, licensed as a treatment for osteoporosis in the UK, but many women with the condition are still not offered it as a treatment choice.

HRT and your heart

Cardiovascular disease is the leading cause of death in women and their risk notably increases after the menopause.[38] The risk of heart attacks is around five times higher after the menopause than before, and heart disease is the leading cause of death for post-menopausal women.[39,40] In addition, heart disease in women is often underdiagnosed, as women can present with different symptoms than men. Plus, the prognosis after a heart attack in a woman is worse than in men.

Typically, women are around ten years older than men when they are first diagnosed with heart disease and this is likely to be related to the decline in hormone levels during the perimeno-pause and menopause.[41] Studies have also shown that women who experience frequent vasomotor symptoms (hot flushes and night sweats) are more likely to develop heart disease and stroke compared to those who do not.[42]

Studies have shown that women who have a later menopause have a lower future risk of heart disease than those who are younger when they become menopausal. This is because the older women have longer with oestrogen in their bodies.[43] Oestrogen and testosterone have important functions in the function of the lining of your blood vessels, the muscular tone of your blood vessels and also the function of your heart.[44,45] Oestrogen allows your blood vessels to relax and widen, so that blood can flow through them easily, which helps to regulate blood pressure. The drop in oestrogen that happens during the menopause may raise your blood pressure, and this is linked to a much higher risk of heart disease and heart attacks.

Oestrogen also acts as an anti-inflammatory in the lining of your blood vessels and increases levels of various chemicals that help to protect your cardiovascular system from disease, such as nitrous oxide and prostacyclin.[46]

Also, when oestrogen falls, the cholesterol in your blood often rises, which can also increase future risk of heart disease. Taking body-identical HRT usually lowers cholesterol – oestrogen can decrease low-density lipoprotein (LDL) cholesterol and increase 'good' high-density lipoprotein (HDL) cholesterol.[47]

By correcting the hormone deficiency and replacing the missing hormones, HRT helps to lower your risk of heart disease in future. Oestrogen reduces inflammation in the endothelium (the lining of the blood vessels), leading to less atheroma developing, which reduces risk of heart disease in the future. Body-identical HRT can also lower blood pressure and reduce the risk of heart failure and also atrial fibrillation occurring. Women who start HRT during the perimenopause or within ten years of the menopause have been shown to have a significantly lower risk of developing heart disease compared to women who don't take it.[48,49] (Women who start taking HRT more than ten years after the menopause are also likely to have a lower future risk of heart disease, but the evidence is less robust.)

The use of other treatments for heart-disease prevention, including statins, has not been shown to be beneficial in women, whereas improving lifestyle can reduce death from heart disease by around 12–14 per cent.[50] However, studies have consistently shown that the risk of dying from heart disease in women taking HRT is reduced by about 30 per cent. This finding is based on data from the Women's Health Initiative in women aged 50–59 years, a Cochrane meta-analysis and another meta-analysis.[51,52,53]

There is a crucial need for more healthcare professionals to be aware of the significant effect the menopause can have on heart-disease risk and the important protective role hormone replacement can have on lowering this.[54]

Spotlight on Blood Pressure

If you're a fan of TV hospital dramas, you're probably used to shouts of 'BP 120 over 80' over the sound of beeping machines and the clatter of medical trolleys. But keeping an eye on blood pressure isn't just a dramatic device – it's a good idea in real life as well.

You can ask for a blood-pressure check if you're worried about it at any time. People over forty can have a blood-pressure test as part of the NHS Health Check, which is offered to forty–seventy-year-olds every five years. However, if you've had high or low blood pressure in the past, or are at risk of developing high blood pressure, you may need to have it checked more frequently.

You would usually have your blood pressure checked at your family doctor or local pharmacy. Blood-pressure monitors vary, but most will work via a cuff secured around your upper arm and then give a digital reading.

Beware of white-coat hypertension

When you visit a surgery or pharmacy, you may get what my medical colleagues call 'white-coat hypertension', whereby feeling a bit anxious or stressed about the test itself can cause your blood pressure to rise. If this happens, don't be embarrassed; it happens more often than you think, but the test only takes a minute. It's important to sit up straight, try to relax and not to talk during the test to get an accurate reading.

What do the numbers mean?

Blood pressure is measured in millimetres of mercury (mmHg) and is given as two numbers: systolic – the pressure when your heart pushes blood out; and diastolic – the pressure when your heart rests between beats. Systolic pressure is always given first.

A normal blood pressure is considered to be between 90/60mmHg and 120/80mmHg (90 over 60 or 120 over 80). High blood pressure is 140/90mmHg or higher; low blood pressure is 90/60mmHg or lower. A reading of between 120/80mmHg and 140/90mmHg is deemed at risk of developing high blood pressure.[55]

Should I buy a home blood-pressure monitor?

Always consult a healthcare professional on whether you need to monitor your blood pressure at home. There are lots of home monitors on the market, and price and quality can vary. If you have been advised to buy one, the British Heart Foundation has an excellent guide on models to buy and how to check your blood pressure at home (see Resources, p. 358).

HRT and diabetes

The incidence of diabetes globally is increasing as the population ages. The menopause is a cardiometabolic condition, meaning that biochemical changes occur in your body when oestrogen levels are low, resulting in metabolic changes such as increased insulin resistance, abdominal-fat occurrence, risk of metabolic syndrome and also risk of type 2 diabetes. In addition, low oestrogen levels can affect insulin production by your pancreas, which also increases future risk of type 2 diabetes.[56,57]

Women who take HRT have a lower future risk of developing type 2 diabetes. This is due to many beneficial effects of oestrogen, including reducing insulin resistance, improving insulin sensitivity in the liver, muscle and fat cells and insulin production in the pancreas.

HRT and bowel cancer

A significant (20 per cent) lower future risk of developing bowel cancer has been shown in women who take HRT.[58] As no other treatment has been developed to prevent bowel cancer, this is an important yet often overlooked finding.[59] Clearly, more research needs to be undertaken in this area.

HRT and death

A prolonged period without oestrogen increases the risk of an earlier death. Clearly, lifestyle and other factors are important, but the beneficial effects of oestrogen have often been forgotten and overlooked over the past twenty years since the launch of the WHI (Women's Health Initiative) study. A 2022 study examining whether HRT had any effect on mortality rates found that women who took combined HRT had a 9 per cent lower risk of death from any cause than non-HRT users.[60]

HRT and other conditions

As mentioned earlier, oestrogen is important for your immune system to work properly and effectively. There are oestrogen receptors on every immune cell and in the presence of oestrogen these cells can work more efficiently, increase in number and also produce different cytokines (chemical substances to protect the body).[61] Diseases associated with inflammation can increase when oestrogen levels are low during the menopause, but these are less likely and also less severe in women who take HRT. They include osteoarthritis, rheumatoid arthritis, multiple sclerosis, Parkinson's disease, leg ulcers, cancer and different infections, including COVID.

EXPERT VIEW
Can HRT reduce your risk of dementia? – neuroscientist Dr Lisa Mosconi PhD,
Director of the Women's Brain Initiative
and author of *The XX Brain*

Lisa is a neuroscientist and author who is doing incredible work highlighting the key issue of brain health and the menopause – a hugely under-researched and underfunded area.

Many of us worry about dementia, particularly if there is someone in our family who has been affected. As there isn't a known cure for dementia, many doctors and scientists focus on prevention, by taking steps to improve heart, metabolic and hormonal health, and reducing known risk factors, which include high blood pressure, diabetes, obesity and smoking.

In recent years, there has been a great deal of research into dementia, and some studies suggest that HRT could potentially reduce the risk, specifically of Alzheimer's, along with other neurodegenerative diseases, including Parkinson's.[62]

Worldwide, women with dementia outnumber men by nearly two to one. It's not yet fully understood why this is the case, and it isn't entirely explained by the fact that women live longer than men. It is important to note that even though the risk of dementia increases with age, it is caused by diseases in the brain and not by age alone.

There is limited knowledge about women's brains and the risk of dementia, partly due to the fact that women have only been included in clinical trials since 1993. However, brain scans indicate that the rate at which brain cells die may be faster in women than in men, and some researchers believe that this could be linked to declining levels of the hormone oestrogen during the perimenopause and menopause. Preclinical studies have shown that oestrogen can have a protective effect on brain cells, which is why researchers are working to assess whether taking HRT could reduce the risk of dementia.[63,64]

The menopause can be a turning point for brain health and cognitive function: oestrogen stimulates the brain, keeps the neurons firing, supports the growth of new cells and helps existing cells to form new connections. When oestrogen levels fall during the menopause transition, your entire body – including your brain – is impacted by this change. We have found that there is an overall reduction of brain-energy levels during the transition to menopause, which might be one reason why you can suffer hot flushes, night sweats, anxiety, depression, brain fog and even memory lapses.

A lot of people see menopause as a natural process we go through, which is absolutely correct. But they don't see it as a process that may increase your risk of future conditions – including dementia – and this is what's really key.

The benefits of HRT

As oestrogen supports brain function, there's increasing evidence to suggest that taking HRT could also play a key role in reducing the risk of dementia. Observational research from the University of Arizona Center for Innovation in Brain Science found that women who took HRT in midlife went on to have a 58 per cent lower risk of Alzheimer's.[65] Taking body-identical HRT (rather than synthetic hormones) resulted in the greatest reduction of risk. HRT administered through the skin in a patch, gel or spray reduced the risk of Alzheimer's, while taking oral HRT (a pill) reduced the risk of combined neurodegenerative diseases.

Taking HRT for more than one year gave greater protection from Alzheimer's, dementia and Parkinson's disease than short-term treatment (where HRT was taken for less than one year). As other studies have shown no protective effects of HRT, more research is urgently needed.

Reducing your risk of dementia

It's crucial to look at lifestyle factors that support brain health to help minimise your risk of dementia. These include eating a healthy diet, taking regular exercise, prioritising relaxation and reducing your stress levels and getting enough sleep.

Timeout #1: Would I benefit from taking HRT?

Take a few minutes to ask yourself the following:

- Do you have symptoms that are affecting your day-to-day life?
- Have you considered how you will safeguard your health in the long term?

When is the best time to start taking HRT?

This is something I get asked about a lot. You don't have to wait until you are menopausal. HRT can be started while you are perimenopausal and, for the majority of women, the benefits outweigh any risks.[66] Research has shown that the earlier a woman starts taking HRT, the better for her future health. However, no one is too old to consider starting HRT.

Timeout #2: Finding the right type of HRT for you

Take a few minutes to consider the following:
- What symptoms are bothering you? Are there any future health concerns that are worrying you?
- What are the main reasons why you would like to take HRT?
- Do you have any health conditions or family medical history to take into account, such as a history of migraines, blood clots or a history of breast cancer?
- Do you still have a uterus?
- Gather information on the different forms of HRT – a patch, spray or gel, for example.

Getting started: How and when to take your HRT – and temporary side effects to be aware of

Trying a new medication can be a bit daunting, especially when, as in the case of HRT, it comes in so many different forms. Am I applying my gel correctly? Have I rubbed it in enough? How long do I leave it to dry? Why isn't my patch sticking? These are just some of the questions I am asked in clinic and on social media on almost a daily basis.

So whether you use gels, sprays, patches or cream, here's the lowdown on how and when to use HRT and any initial side effects you might experience.

Gel

Gel is licensed for use on your arms or thighs. However, it can usually be used on other areas of the body, too. It's best to rub it in, rather than leaving it to dry naturally – about the same amount of time as you would spend applying a body moisturiser will suffice. Once the gel is absorbed, you can wear clothes and exercise normally, although it is usually sensible to wait for about half an hour before applying sunscreen or moisturiser.

Spray

Spray should usually be used on the inner part of your forearm.

Patches

Patches should be put on the skin below your waist – most people stick them on their bottom, upper thigh or lower back. After applying, smooth over to make sure there are no air bubbles and place your hand over the patch for a few seconds to warm it and ensure it adheres to your skin.

Testosterone cream or gel
Testosterone is usually rubbed into the lower abdomen, the skin of your buttock or on your thigh.

When should I use HRT?
It's better to use your gel or spray after a shower or swimming. Always wash your hands afterwards and wait for an hour before letting anyone else touch the areas where you have applied the gel or spray, so that it is fully absorbed.

Do I have to use my dose of gel or spray in one go?
Most women will be prescribed two to four pumps of gel or spray a day. If that feels like a lot in one go, you can space it out – for example, half in the morning and half before going to bed.

Will my patch stay in place?
Patches are usually changed twice a week, so they should stay in place for three or four days, including in the shower or bath. If you have trouble making them stick, a quick wipe of surgical spirit on the skin before applying should help. If they are still not sticking well, you should try either an alternative patch or a different type of oestrogen, such as the gel.

Do I need to take my HRT at the same time every day?
It's helpful to get into a routine, so you remember to take/apply your HRT as directed. How that routine works is entirely up to you: you might have more time in the evening to apply gels,

creams and patches, or you might want to get it all done during your morning routine. Take micronised progesterone in the evening, as it has a mild sedative effect, so it can help you sleep – and remember, it ideally needs to be taken on an empty stomach.

You would normally look to take your HRT at the same time each day, but the odd hour's difference here and there won't matter; what is more important is that you are taking the amount prescribed for you, as directed by your healthcare professional, on a consistent basis.

If it is a split dose, must the doses be exactly twelve hours apart?

Twelve hours is a rough guideline, but it isn't essential – busy lives and memory slips mean you might not always take it at the twelve-hour mark. Try to aim for twelve-hour intervals, but a few hours either side shouldn't present a problem.

Just started taking HRT? Remember the four Bs

Starting a new medication can be daunting, and HRT is no different. Getting used to a new routine and remembering to use your treatments at the right time can be a challenge, while noticing new side effects can also be a cause for concern.

During the early weeks, women will often mistake temporary side effects as a sign their HRT isn't working, when, in actual fact, they need to give it some time to get to work. HRT can often take several weeks or even months before the positive effects are fully felt.

Whenever you start a new treatment, you should always be aware of the difference between what can be considered a normal side effect and symptoms that might require a follow-up with your healthcare professional. To help my patients remember the common side effects that can occur during the first few weeks after starting HRT, I tell them to learn the four Bs:

1. **Bleeding.** This could be a brown discharge, light spotting or sometimes more like a heavy period and may come and go or last for a few weeks. Any bleeding should usually settle down after a few weeks, but if you are experiencing it for more than three months after starting HRT, contact your healthcare professional. You do not need to stop taking your HRT if you experience bleeding.

2. **Breasts.** Your breasts may become tender, be quite painful and more sensitive around the nipples. This can last for several weeks, but usually settles with time. Wearing a well-fitting, supportive bra can help with tenderness and pain, but, if it does not settle, the dose or type of HRT may need to be changed.

3. **Bloating.** Progesterone or synthetic progestogens can cause an uncomfortable, bloated feeling, but this should settle down with time.

4. **The Blues.** You might find you suffer from low mood or are more tearful in the first few weeks of HRT (or more emotional if you're taking progesterone, such as Utrogestan). This usually improves but, if it does not, you should consider changing the type of progesterone.

All these symptoms should usually settle down within three months of taking your HRT so, if it has only been a week or two, try to stick with it and wait and see. If you're still troubled by

111

side effects after three months, discuss them with your health-care professional.

Symptoms still not improving?

Don't give up. For some women it can take many months to find the right dose and type of HRT that really works for them.

Your healthcare professional may have given you a range within which to manage the dose yourself – for example, 'one to three pumps' of oestrogen gel. You can alter the dose your-self within the range prescribed for you, but just remember – your body can take a few weeks to respond to any changes you make.

And remember also that there are so many different types and ways to take HRT. So if you don't feel your HRT has brought you the benefits you were hoping for after three months, discuss with your healthcare professional whether you can change the dose or the way you take the medication. Some women find that adding testosterone to their HRT really improves their persistent symptoms.

EXPERT VIEW
Can I take HRT while breastfeeding? – Dr Wendy Jones,
Pharmacist with a special interest in the safety of drugs in breast milk and founder of website www.breastfeeding-and-medication.co.uk

A community pharmacist by background, Wendy works to raise awareness and knowledge around breastfeeding and medication through her website, and on e-learning materials for healthcare professionals and parents.

Growing awareness that perimenopause and menopause symptoms can start in your mid-to-late thirties and early forties, when you may still be fertile and having periods, has led to an increase in people seeking treatment like HRT earlier than ever before.

We are also starting families later in life – the average age of first-time mums in England and Wales in 2020 was 30.7 years, up from 26.4 years in 1974.[67]

Different phases of our lives don't neatly stop and then another one starts, so, while less common, it is possible to become pregnant during the menopause. In addition, if you choose to breast-feed your child for more than a year, it is possible you may reach the point where you become perimenopausal or menopausal while you are still breastfeeding.

Access to effective and safe treatment for your perimenopause or menopause if you have recently given birth or are breastfeeding can be challenging. Oestrogen levels drop after childbirth and during breastfeeding, which can result in symptoms that often mimic those experienced during the perimenopause, such as hot flushes and night sweats, headaches or joint pains. Psychological symptoms, such as low mood and irritability and trouble sleeping are also familiar features in the postnatal period for many reasons. Hence mothers may be treated for depression, rather than investigated for perimenopause.

Healthcare professionals' understanding of perimenopausal symptoms can be limited, and more so if you are breastfeeding as well, particularly outside of the perceived 'normal' timeframe.

So with this in mind, it's helpful to keep track of your periods (if you have them) and log all your symptoms in preparation for an appointment with your healthcare professional.

HRT and breastfeeding: what you need to know

HRT contains the hormones oestrogen and a progesterone (if you still have your uterus). These are similar to the hormones found in the combined oral contraceptive pill, which we know can be safely used while breastfeeding.

In comparison to the combined contraceptive pill, HRT contains much lower amounts of these hormones, and body-identical HRT (transdermal oestrogen and micronised progesterone) mimics the natural hormones that your body produces.

There is little research on the passage of HRT into breast milk, but, anecdotally, many women continue to take it without it impacting their baby or breast-milk supply. The decision on whether to take HRT should be yours, after a discussion with a healthcare professional.

Using vaginal HRT while breastfeeding

Breastfeeding can affect natural vaginal lubrication so vaginal dryness can become a particular problem for those who are already in the perimenopause. Local oestrogen (which is placed directly into the vagina) may be prescribed when breastfeeding, usually to help with the healing of stitches after childbirth, prolapses or ongoing vaginal dryness.

If over-the-counter vaginal moisturisers don't provide relief, it can be very effective to deliver oestrogen straight to the affected area with vaginal oestrogen.

Can you start HRT at any age?

Is there a cut-off age for starting HRT? If you have been taking it for years, when should you think about stopping it? These questions are often asked by women who have had their menopause some time ago.

Some women just take HRT for a few years to help improve the worst symptoms of their menopause. Some find that when they stop taking HRT after just a few years, they have no more symptoms; others experience a return when they stop.

However, increasingly, women are taking HRT to improve their future health.

Simply put, there is no set length of time you should take HRT for. Because the menopause is a long-term hormone deficiency it means that women can usually take it for ever to replace these missing hormones.

Many women are not prescribed HRT at the point when they develop symptoms of the menopause, usually due to unfounded fears about perceived risks. This also may be because their symptoms weren't too bad, or they felt they had to simply grin and bear it. Or they may have had significant concerns over the safety of HRT, or other healthcare professionals may have advised against it.

You might be reading this book, wondering if you can revisit a decision you made years ago, as HRT is now becoming a more attractive option for you.

There is very little good-quality evidence regarding women over sixty starting HRT for the first time because this research has not been undertaken. However, in my clinical experience, most women who are otherwise fit and well do usually still gain some benefits from taking HRT – even if it has been ten years since their menopause.

You may decide to start HRT now because your symptoms have worsened, or you were expecting them to have gone by now but they haven't. You may be concerned about the long-term risks associated with the low levels of hormones that occur during the menopause in later life – such as the risk of cardiovascular disease and osteoporosis, as well as diabetes, dementia and depression. These are all valid reasons for wanting to take HRT at this point in your life.

It is important that you seek individualised advice from your doctor or another healthcare professional and discuss all the treatment options available to you. If your regular doctor or healthcare professional will not consider HRT for you, you may wish to find a doctor or nurse who has a special interest in the menopause, so that you can have a more detailed discussion with them.

I stopped taking HRT some time ago. Can I start again?

You may be someone who has previously taken HRT but stopped, either by choice or reluctantly, after being advised to by a healthcare professional. If you want to start again, see another healthcare professional to explain your reasons. The NICE guidelines are clear that women can continue to take HRT for as long as the benefits outweigh the risks. Many women can safely restart HRT, and the body-identical HRT with oestrogen through the skin as a patch, gel or spray is usually preferable.

HRT risks in perspective

....

For the vast majority of women, the benefits of HRT far outweigh the risks. Yet many are reluctant to take it. And some of those who *do* want to take it can encounter resistance from healthcare professionals.

One block to women getting help – and relief from symptoms – is that nagging doubt that HRT is too risky and causes breast cancer, which is incorrect.

Let's take some time to fully explore where the rumours come from and have a look at the evidence.

As part of the feminist movement in the 1960s, the idea of 'feminine forever' was introduced in a bestselling book of the same name by an American doctor – Robert Wilson. He was among the first to recognise that the hormone deficiency that occurs during perimenopause and menopause could be prevented and corrected with oestrogen replacement.

In the US and Europe, HRT grew in popularity over the decades, rising significantly in the 1990s. The majority of menopausal women took HRT, and healthcare professionals were very happy and willing to prescribe it.

But in the early 2000s, everything changed. In 1993, the Women's Health Initiative (WHI) had begun a clinical trial looking at the health effects of women taking oestrogen-only or combined HRT compared to a placebo. The type of HRT used in this study contained oestrogen derived from pregnant horses' urine and a synthetic progestogen; this is very different from the body-identical HRT we now usually prescribe, which has lower risks and is very safe. And in 2002, the combined HRT part of the study was halted prematurely, due to results linking HRT with breast cancer, heart disease, stroke and blood clots.

The conclusions were then leaked to the lay and medical press without the results being properly analysed first. Yet later analysis of the data revealed the link with breast cancer was not statistically significant – in fact, oestrogen-only HRT was subsequently shown to be associated with a *lower* risk of breast cancer – but the damage was done. The notion that all HRT caused breast cancer was now firmly planted in the minds of women and healthcare professionals alike.

As a result, numbers of women taking HRT worldwide fell sharply.

A deep dive into the WHI study found the following:[68]

- The average age of women in the study was sixty-three, yet researchers wrongly generalised their conclusions to include women entering menopause in their early fifties.
- Nearly half the participants were current or past smokers, many had had heart disease in the past, more than a third had been treated for high blood pressure, and 70 per cent were seriously overweight or obese.
- The study claimed HRT increased the risk of heart problems, but the proper analysis revealed that the risk occurred only among women who were starting it in their seventies and older.
- The investigators revised their findings five years after they were initially published and concluded that women who started HRT in the first ten years following the beginning of menopause actually reduced their risk of heart disease – but this didn't make headlines either.
- Further analysis of the study showed that there was a

significantly lower risk of breast cancer in women who took oestrogen-only HRT (so those women who'd had a hysterectomy in the past) and a lower risk of dying from breast cancer in women who took any type of HRT.

- The risk of breast cancer in women taking HRT with synthetic progestogen was very small and not even statistically significant.
- There was a lower risk of developing colon cancer in women who took HRT.

The benefits of HRT usually far outweigh any risks, and body-identical HRT containing oestrogen in the form of 17 beta-oestradiol and micronised progesterone is extremely safe. The risks of HRT depend on the type you are given and other factors, such as your age, weight, alcohol intake and whether you smoke. This is why it is so important to have an individualised consultation, where you can discuss *your* actual risks.

Risk of blood clot
You are more likely to develop a clot or have a stroke if you are obese, a smoker or have had a clot in the past.

There is a small increased risk of a clot or stroke if you take oestrogen in tablet form. To understand how small this risk is, imagine a healthy fifty-year-old woman who has a VTE (venous thromboembolism – a term referring to blood clots in the veins) risk of around 6 in 10,000 per year; if she took oestrogen tablets, this would double her risk to around 12 in 10,000, but it's still a small risk overall. Oestrogen via a patch, gel or spray does not carry an increased risk of clot or stroke.[69] This type of HRT is also safe for women to take, even if they have a high risk of clot or have had one in the past.[70] This is because oestrogen used in this way goes straight into your bloodstream, so bypasses the liver, which produces your clotting factors. When oestrogen is taken orally, it is metabolised in the liver, so stimulates the clotting factors.

Risk of breast cancer

It can be common for people to worry about breast cancer when taking HRT. Most types do not actually increase the risk of breast cancer. The only type that might have a very small risk is HRT containing both oestrogen and the *older* synthetic types of progestogen. And this is only if you're over fifty-one years of age. The risk is related to the type of progestogen in the HRT and not the oestrogen – taking micronised progesterone (the body-identical progesterone) has not been shown in studies to have an increased risk of breast cancer.

Even if you're over fifty-one years and take the synthetic type, such as combined HRT patches, the risk is very low. In fact, the risk is less than the increased risk if you drink a couple of glasses of wine each night or the increased risk of being overweight.

The risk or perceived risk of breast cancer with HRT is the biggest reason why women are scared to take HRT and why women refuse to be prescribed HRT.

Unfortunately, unwarranted mistrust and fear of HRT have become deeply rooted and prevail among health practitioners, women, and the media.[71]

Any risks of HRT should be put in context. Benefits of HRT should be discussed and considered. Women should be pivotal in the decision-making process.

Preventing a woman from the benefits of HRT is resulting in millions of women having menopausal symptoms and having adverse effects on their heart, bone, mood, sexual health, and cognition.

And it's worth bearing in mind that there has never been a study showing that women who take HRT have a higher risk of dying from breast cancer. There does not seem to be an increased risk of breast cancer when using the Mirena coil.

If you've had a hysterectomy and are taking oestrogen without a progestogen, you actually have a lower risk of developing breast cancer than someone who doesn't take HRT at all.[72]

Finally, all the evidence has shown that women taking any type of HRT (oestrogen only or combined HRT) have a lower risk of dying from breast cancer compared to women who have not taken it.[73,74]

CASE STUDY: HRT GAVE ME MY
LIFE BACK – ANONYMOUS

One of the most rewarding aspects of being known for menopause care and awareness is when I receive messages from women (and their partners and children) saying that advice or words of encouragement I've offered have had a positive impact on their lives. Often, these are from patients, but sometimes they will come from a woman who has taken the time to read one of my social media posts, listened to a podcast or used the balance app.

An anonymous email, which landed in my inbox a while ago, is one such rewarding note. And for me, these messages are so very special because they encapsulate exactly what I set out to achieve in those early years of my first website: a place for women to find out more, read the latest research and feel empowered and supported. Though not a patient of mine, she had followed me on social media and had accessed my balance website for menopause advice.

Her message was so eloquently written, and her story was so vivid that the words practically leapt off the page.

Here was a woman, like so many others, who had faced multiple healthcare appointments and prescriptions for various medications before it emerged she was menopausal.

She described her menopause journey and the symptoms that had affected her career, her finances and relationships with those closest to her.

After reading up on the menopause and persevering with healthcare professionals, she said the turning point was HRT.

'I just needed my hormones back,' she wrote, excitedly telling me about new career prospects, growing confidence and self-esteem, a renewed social life and the joy of spending time with her loved ones.

It was a joy to read how hormones had given her back her zest for life, and how she was now looking to help others in similar situations by recommending my website and app.

The email ended with the woman thanking me for campaigning for better menopause education and spoke of the need to pave the way for future generations.

This woman will never know, but her email arrived in my inbox at exactly the right time.

Testosterone: what is it – and do I need it?

Testosterone is a biologically active hormone that is important for many women. There are cells that respond to testosterone all over the body, and levels gradually decline with age in women. Symptoms of testosterone deficiency can include fatigue, loss of concentration, impaired memory, brain fog, reduced energy, headaches, low mood, loss of muscle strength and reduced libido.[75]

Current UK NHS guidelines only recommend testosterone if you have severely reduced libido or hypoactive sexual desire disorder (see box),[76] but there is increasing evidence to show that the benefits of testosterone could help many more women in their perimenopause and menopause.

Many menopause specialists, and increasingly GPs, are realising the widespread benefits of testosterone replacement for most women. Benefits of testosterone can include improved muscle mass and strength, enhanced concentration, clarity of thought and memory and better sleep.[77]

When would testosterone be considered?

There is no wrong or right time to start testosterone. More study needs to be undertaken in this area, and we are already doing some exciting research into it with a team of people.

You do not usually need to have a blood test before treatment is started; your symptoms are usually enough of a guide for your healthcare professional to agree to prescribe testosterone. It is possible to measure your testosterone levels in your blood by having your total testosterone and sex hormone binding globulin (SHBG) levels checked and your free androgen index (FAI) calculated. This can be a useful test to assess your response to treatment with testosterone. Your clinician is likely to want to do these tests a few months and then annually after starting treatment with testosterone to ensure your levels are within the 'female' range.

What is hypoactive sexual desire disorder?

Menopause or no menopause, it's completely normal to go through phases of being less interested in sex. Tiredness, stress, life and bodily changes like weight gain, night sweats or aches and pains can put even the most physical relationships under strain. And the fact that so few women talk about the impact it has on their sex lives can make the problem even worse.

But there is a key difference between 'not tonight' and 'no, never'. When that disinterest becomes more than a phase and a permanent state of being, then you may have hypoactive sexual desire disorder (HSDD). This is deemed to be a total lack of interest, lasting for more than six months, that has consequences on your relationship and/or self-esteem.

Common symptoms of HSDD include:

· no interest in any type of sexual activity
· no sexual thoughts or fantasies
· no interest in initiating sex
· not being responsive to stimulation or difficulty gaining pleasure, including masturbation.

One paper put the prevalence of HSDD at about 8.9 per cent of women aged eighteen to forty-four, 12.3 per cent of forty-five- to sixty-four-year-olds, and 7.4 per cent in women over sixty-five.[78]

Here are some of the questions that are asked when a diagnosis of HSDD is considered:

- In the past, was your level of sexual desire or interest good and satisfying to you?
- Has there been a decrease in your level of sexual desire or interest?
- Does your decreased level of sexual desire or interest bother you?
- Would you like your level of sexual desire or interest to increase?
- What are the factors that you feel contribute to your current decrease in sexual desire or interest (this could include depression, a medical condition or surgery, medication, drugs or alcohol, pregnancy, recent childbirth or menopause, sexual issues, such as pain or decreased arousal or relationship difficulties)?

A lack of libido doesn't have to be an inevitable consequence of getting older, and you can speak to someone about it. There's no one test for HSDD but speak to a healthcare professional and explain how your low sex drive is impacting you and any relationships you have. They will want to explore the root cause, which can often be a combination of factors. Then, depending on the cause, you can look to make some positive changes. This might be HRT including testosterone, vaginal oestrogen if sex is uncomfortable, changing other medications you might be on that are lowering your libido, psychosexual counselling for yourself or as a couple.

And there are also some simple changes to routines that can help to relieve stress and improve intimacy, such as exercising regularly to boost self-esteem, taking part in activities you both find relaxing, planning times for connection and intimacy, sexual experimentation (this could include different positions, places, role play or sex toys) and avoiding substances like tobacco and alcohol that can reduce sexual desire and performance.

In addition, systemic transdermal testosterone is recommended for women with HSDD who do not have any modifiable factors or contributory conditions, such as relationship or mental-health problems.[79]

How is testosterone treatment given?

Testosterone is usually given as a cream or gel (in the UK, it is available as AndroFeme®1 cream, Testogel® or Testim® gel), which you rub into your skin like a moisturiser, and it's then absorbed directly into your bloodstream. AndroFeme®1 is made for women and is a regulated preparation, while Testogel® and Tostran® gels are made for men but can be safely used in lower doses for women, as it is the same hormone.

Testosterone is usually given with HRT. Many women start taking testosterone a few months or so after starting HRT, but some choose to start it at the same time. Some also take testosterone without HRT, but this is less common.

Your clinician will tell you how much to use. It should be rubbed on to clean, dry skin on your upper outer thigh or buttocks and usually takes about thirty seconds to dry. Try to apply at the same time each day to establish a routine, and always wash your hands thoroughly after using it. Avoid swimming or showering for around thirty minutes after application.

Some menopause specialists give testosterone as an implant, which is a tiny pellet inserted under your skin and usually stays there for six months.

How long before I notice a difference?

It can sometimes take a few months for the full effects of testosterone to work in your body, whether this is using the cream, gel or the implant.

Using testosterone cream or gel daily will help to restore your blood testosterone levels back into the normal range for you and many women notice that it can also often improve tiredness, brain fog and low sex drive, among other things.

You should usually have a blood test to check your testosterone levels after around three months, and you should be reviewed by your doctor three to six months after starting treatment and then annually.

What about side effects?

This can be something women are concerned about with testosterone. There are usually no side effects when testosterone is prescribed properly and you are simply replacing the missing amount, so your levels are still within normal range for women. Very rarely, women notice some increased hair growth in the actual area where the cream has been applied. You can avoid this happening by rubbing the cream or gel into places where you have fewer hair follicles (such as the upper outer thighs and buttocks) and by regularly changing the area of skin where you apply it.

As the dose is so low, testosterone used in this way does not usually increase your risk of developing facial hair, voice deepening or skin changes. It is important to have regular (usually annual) blood monitoring to reduce the risk of any side effects.

Testosterone can be taken safely alongside oestrogen HRT and vaginal oestrogen. Long-term use of safely prescribed testosterone replacement is not associated with any adverse health effects.

Note: AndroFeme®1 contains almond oil, so should not be used if you have an allergy to almonds.

CASE STUDY: TESTOSTERONE
AND ME – YVE'S STORY

When it comes to describing the impact testosterone can have, I think it only fair to hand over to Yve. Already on HRT, but finding her libido had not improved, Yve happened upon an article on testosterone. She's been taking it since 2017 and says it has changed her sex life for the better.

'I first read about testosterone as a treatment for low sex drive in an article on how the actress Jane Fonda used it.[80] When I read the article, I was massively relieved to hear of similar symptoms to my own. She described feeling increasingly emotionally remote from her husband, despite taking HRT. She felt there must be another cause and had found discussions around testosterone.

'I found myself feeling revolted by intimate advances from my husband, but at the same time appalled by those feelings, particularly as I had been formerly very happy about sex and gone on to HRT in my late forties to try and address a lowered libido. It fixed the functionality of a shrunken vagina and vaginal dryness but didn't help with sexual feeling or ability to orgasm. I felt that any sexual feeling was switched off. Disconnected.

'I saw a specialist. She prescribed testosterone for five years with a review after the first three months. I use the recommended one 50g sachet over a week. In fact, I need less than that over the long term.

'I found it life-changing. I discovered that subtle sensations reappeared. It brought back connection with my clitoral sensation and so orgasms resumed reliably. I found my husband sexy again and someone I could relax with. The negativity definitely creeps back in again if I don't take it for more than ten days.

'I'm sure testosterone could be an enormous leap forward for many women. Not everyone wants to keep going with sexual activity, but many women might underestimate the effect on their intimate relationships of not being in step with a sexual partner and of having strong feelings of unpleasantness around intimacy. They might like to have the choice.

'I have found it a difficult subject to raise with my best friends in my old antenatal group. People are very embarrassed and must feel they just have to get over that part of their lives. It needs exploration, though.

'I suppose I don't need to go on being sexually active for ever, but I do want to remain in step with my husband.'

Vaginal hormones

Systemic HRT medicines circulate in the blood and can be administered by oral tablets, patches and skin gels and spray. Vaginal hormones are different to systemic HRT, but I have included it in this chapter because it is very often used alongside HRT. Vaginal hormonal treatments can also be used on their own, without HRT.

As I covered earlier in this book, vulval, vaginal and urinary symptoms associated with the perimenopause and menopause can be particularly distressing menopause symptoms; they often worsen with time and usually persist for ever.[81] Despite GSM being very common and often having a very negative effect on women's quality of life, it is still underdiagnosed and often not treated or treated too late.[82] Often, patients will respond very well to HRT, but symptoms associated with vaginal dryness and urinary symptoms can still be an issue.

However, the good news is that there are really effective treatments for these symptoms that can be taken alongside systemic HRT or used on their own. A very effective solution is to put oestrogen directly on the affected area. This is known as 'local' or 'topical' oestrogen, and is not the same as the oestrogen you take as part of your HRT; vaginal-oestrogen treatments can be taken safely for a long time (usually for ever), with no associated risks.[83]

How do I use it?

There are two types of oestrogen used – oestradiol and oestriol – and three main ways to absorb it directly from your vagina and surrounding area:

- **Pessary:** the most common choice of vaginal oestrogen is a pessary, such as Vagifem® (containing oestradiol). This is a small tablet you insert into your vagina, using an applicator. It is administered daily for the first two weeks, and then twice weekly after that. Women usually insert the pessary at night, so it can stay in place in your vagina for several hours. If twice weekly doesn't improve symptoms, it can be used more frequently under advice from your healthcare professional.

Imvaggis® pessaries are a more gentle, lower-dose alternative and contain oestriol. They look like small, waxy bullets and do not require an applicator for insertion, so are more environmentally friendly. They can, however, sometimes result in a discharge when the product dissolves and leaves your vagina. Women use one pessary every night for three weeks, then twice a week thereafter. There is another type of pessary that is different to other oestrogen preparations: Intrarosa®, containing DHEA, a hormone that our bodies naturally produce. Once positioned in your vagina, the DHEA is converted to both oestrogen and testosterone.[84] It can be used with or without an applicator and the usual dose is one pessary every night.

- **Cream or gel:** oestrogen creams, such as Ovestin® (containing estriol), are inserted inside the vagina on a daily basis for the first fortnight, and then twice weekly after that. An applicator can be used to insert the cream in your vagina, or it can be applied with the fingertips on and around your vulva area as well – which can be useful if you are experiencing itching or soreness of your external genitalia, too.

Blissel® gel is a newer product that also contains oestriol. This is a lower-dose option (but not quite as low as Imvaggis®) and it has an applicator to insert the gel inside your vagina. It is used every night for three weeks, then twice a week after that.

- **Ring:** an alternative way to use vaginal oestrogen is with an oestrogen ring, such as Estring®. This is a soft, flexible, silicon ring you insert inside your vagina. The ring's centre releases a slow and steady dose of oestradiol over ninety days and needs to be replaced every three months. A health-care professional can insert the ring if you do not feel confident or able to do so. The dose released is slightly stronger than the Vagifem® pessary. You can leave the ring in position to have sex or can remove and reinsert if preferred.

When will I start to see an improvement?

Your symptoms should improve after about three months of using vaginal oestrogen treatments or moisturisers. Some women see significant improvement using oestradiol-containing products and not with oestriol – for other women, it is vice versa. Many women see good results with either type of oestrogen or with DHEA. It can often be a case of trying a few preparations before finding the one most suitable for you. If you have still not had an improvement after three months, you should see your doctor, as sometimes these symptoms can be due to other conditions. It is also very important to see your doctor if you have any unusual bleeding from your vagina.

Over-the-counter vaginal oestrogen: what you need to know

Since September 2022, post-menopausal women have been able to buy a brand of vaginal oestrogen tablets called Gina, without the need for a prescription. While the change is a great initial step forward, it isn't cheap, and all other forms of vaginal oestrogen and systemic HRT remain prescription-only.

In addition, there are several exclusions on who can access Gina: at the time of writing, only post-menopausal women aged fifty years and over and who have not had a period for at least a year are able to buy it.

And while the medicines watchdog (the Medicines and Healthcare products Regulatory Agency) stresses the risk of side effects from this form of hormonal treatment is very low, some women will still require a prescription.[85] This includes those who have had breast, endometrial or ovarian cancer, blood clots, heart disease, liver disease or stroke.

Any other exclusions to Gina?

Women with a history of endometriosis (where tissue similar to the lining of the womb grows elsewhere in the body) can buy Gina if they have previously had a prescription for vaginal oestrogen and they have had no recent symptoms of the condition.

Women already taking systemic HRT can only buy Gina if they have previously had similar vaginal oestrogen or their GP has confirmed that Gina is a good option for them.

SURVEY: YOUR EXPERIENCES OF HEALTHCARE AND HRT

So how are women accessing menopause care?

My survey looked at your experiences of healthcare appointments and HRT.

It found women most commonly saw their usual GP, followed by a menopause specialist in a dedicated menopause clinic, or another GP at their own surgery.

Experiences of consultations and access to care varied. While one in four (25 per cent) said they had received excellent care from the first healthcare professional they saw, 31 per cent said they had received good care overall, but it had taken 'several months' to access it. Some 18 per cent said they were very disappointed with the level of care from their first consultation.

One in five (20 per cent) said their healthcare professional identified their symptoms may be due to changing hormones at their first appointment, while 30 per cent had to have between two and five different appointments/investigations. Some 9 per cent faced six to ten appointments, while 7 per cent had more than ten appointments.

A very encouraging three in four (79 per cent of respondents) said they were currently taking HRT.

5

Mental Health and Menopause

Four things you will learn in this chapter:

1. How mental health can be affected by the perimenopause and menopause

2. Coping strategies – and why antidepressants won't usually tackle perimenopause- and menopause-related low mood

3. A two-way street: how sleep impacts our mental health, and vice versa

4. Coping with the perimenopause or menopause and existing mental-health conditions

Let's start this chapter with a question: how are you feeling today?

Our tendency in responding to a question like this is to treat it as a casual greeting rather than a genuine question, batting it back to the other person with a swift 'I'm fine, how are you?' But take a few moments to consider what I am asking here; and be honest with yourself: how *are* you feeling, really?

Whenever I do a podcast or post on social media about menopause and mental health, I am absolutely inundated with messages from women, usually asking the same two broad questions: 'What is wrong with me?' followed by, 'Why can't I get any help?'

Fluctuating hormones can have an immense impact on mental health. Previously rock-solid relationships can begin to falter, work may seem insurmountable and activities you previously took pleasure in now feel like a chore.

Many women know something isn't right, but they can't quite put their finger on the root cause. When I was perimenopausal, I'd burst into tears at nothing, then spend the next ten minutes bewildered as to what had set me off in the first place. I also often felt very low in my mood and became more socially withdrawn. I had very low self-esteem and lost much of my self-confidence. Until this time, I had really underestimated the power of my hormones over my mental health.

More often than not, life events other than hormonal changes are used to explain why you feel the way you do. To avoid this, it is vital you know the signs of perimenopause- and menopause-related low mood. Women are two to four times more likely to experience major depression during the perimenopausal or early post-menopausal phase.

At 'best', you may experience no symptoms at all, or subtle mood changes that can be managed with coping strategies like breathing techniques or by talking to loved ones. But at the other end of the scale, the mood changes that can come with the perimenopause and menopause can be life-threatening. Most weeks, my clinic takes a call from a woman who is feeling suicidal, and we keep emergency appointments free so that these women can get access to the help and treatment they need. No one should ever feel like they are left without options when it comes to their mental health.

Later on in this chapter, we will hear from Clair (a GP with a special interest in the menopause) about her own suicidal thoughts, which persisted for some years in the run-up to her periods. It was only when a specialist identified that these feelings were likely due to hormonal changes that she started effective treatment that really improved her symptoms. As she puts it, 'Had I not had this awareness and the means to see a menopause specialist, who knows what the outcome may have been?'

Clair's story shows that with the right treatment, huge improvements can be made. But before we get to that point, the right diagnosis and *appropriate* treatment must be in place. Too often, women are told their symptoms are down to clinical depression and are offered and prescribed antidepressants to try to regulate and improve their moods, which often do not help or work. In this chapter, we will be looking at the distinct differences between the two, so if you do decide to look at treatment options, you are informed about which *are* appropriate – and how to know if you are offered something that is inappropriate.

We will also be looking at different techniques to de-stress and restore a sense of balance at this time, including some simple relaxation exercises and tips on what to do if you feel overwhelmed. Plus, sleep expert Dr David Garley, a GP and managing director of The Better Sleep Clinic, will be sharing how changes to your sleep can affect your mental health, along with some tips on how to improve 'sleep hygiene' – that is, healthy habits to adopt for a better night's sleep.

What's wrong with me? How menopause can affect our moods and mental health

Let's go back to the initial question at the start of this chapter. How have you been feeling lately?

Happy, contented and even-tempered? Or maybe a bit low and demotivated, or anxious, annoyed, depressed or even angry? You might have noticed that these moods come with some physical symptoms like faster or more shallow breathing, or feeling light-headed or nauseous. Or do your moods change quickly, so that you find yourself irritated beyond belief one moment and in floods of tears the next?

All those feelings fall into the bracket of perimenopause- or menopause-related low mood. And the reason? Those three key hormones – oestrogen, progesterone and testosterone – and the part they play in regulating mood.[86]

Oestrogen helps to regulate several hormones with mood-boosting properties, including serotonin, which helps with your mood, energy, motivation and sleep.[87] Oestrogen also can help with cognition, so reduced levels can lead to brain fog and forgetfulness, which can also lower your mood. Oestrogen works in many different areas of your brain, including the hypothalamus, amygdala and hippocampus, which are all important areas to regulate mood.

Oestrogen is known to have protective effects on your brain, and it makes sense that during the perimenopause and

138

menopause, with fluctuating and decreasing levels in the brain, the diminution of its neuroprotective benefits can have negative psychological consequences in some women. Furthermore, the menopause can lead to physical changes, loss of certain bodily functions and changes to feelings of femininity.[88]

Progesterone has a mild sedative effect and can help you to feel calm and relaxed.[89] So when this hormone falls, you may feel more irritable or quicker to anger. And a lack of testosterone can negatively affect memory and mood.[90]

Many women find that psychological symptoms are worse during the perimenopause when hormone levels can wildly fluctuate. These fluctuations can trigger changes in mood – being calm one minute and then angry and irrational the next can be very common during this time.

There is evidence that episodes of depression and low mood associated with reproductive events are also triggered by hormonal fluctuations. This means that reproductive-affective disorders that are associated with mood changes such as PMS, PMDD, postnatal depression and perimenopause- and menopause-related depression are distinct forms of depression and many specialists refer to this as reproductive depression.[91]

This means also that women who have experienced PMS, PMDD and postnatal depression are more likely to experience mood changes during the perimenopause and menopause, as areas of their brains are more sensitive to hormonal changes.

Are my feelings normal or perimenopause- or menopause-related?

As humans it is entirely normal to experience a range of emotions, but if you feel your moods have become more extreme or switch up more frequently, it is worth asking yourself the questions below to see if hormones are the cause. If you can, ask a loved one or close friend the same set of questions about you, and then compare notes to see if they have noticed any changes in you.

- Am I feeling more down/worried/irritable/angry than usual?
- [If you are still having periods] Do these mood changes happen around my period?
- Have these feelings become more intense?
- Are my moods affecting my life in terms of motivation, sleep, eating, exercise?
- Are these moods affecting work and home relationships – are these changes affecting those close to me more than usual?
- Have these mood changes lasted for a few weeks or more?

If you find you have answered yes to the majority of these questions, it may be time to speak to a healthcare professional about some strategies and treatments to help with moods.

Treatment options

Research suggests that women with no history of depression are two to four times more likely to report depressed mood compared with pre-menopausal women.[92] It is therefore important that GPs and other healthcare professionals have an awareness of these symptoms in these women and the possible underlying causes – in particular, hormonal ones. Healthcare professionals may not think of hormones as the primary cause of symptoms for women in their late thirties or early forties, for example, but it is not unusual for menopausal symptoms to start as young as this, even younger, for some women.

HRT

As with other menopause-related symptoms, HRT is usually the first-line treatment in replacing hormones you are lacking, so you can refer back to Chapter 4 for a run-down of the different types and the ways to take it. You should usually expect your psychological symptoms to start levelling out and improving within a few months; however, if you are not seeing much of a difference, speak to your healthcare professional to work out if a different dose, type or method would be better suited to you.

HRT, preferably oestrogen through the skin as a gel, patch or spray, should usually be offered as the first-line treatment to a perimenopausal or menopausal woman with mild perimeno-pausal depressive symptoms.[93] Women with a uterus also need a type of progesterone; however, many women with reproductive depression are sensitive or even intolerant to some types of progesterones (usually the synthetic progestogens that are in the combined oral contraceptive pills and also in older types of HRT).[94] Micronised progesterone (orally or vaginally) and the Mirena coil have been shown to be better tolerated than other progestogens with regard to mood-related side effects.[95]

Cognitive behavioural therapy (CBT)

A type of talking therapy, CBT focuses on breaking unhelpful behavioural patterns and behaviours that we adopt in relation to challenges or stressful situations. It is used for a range of mental and physical health conditions and is recommended in the NICE menopause guidelines as being helpful for menopause-related low mood and anxiety. CBT may also improve sleep and vaso-motor symptoms in some women.[96]

CBT is usually delivered one to one. You will likely be asked to focus on your thoughts, feelings and attitudes and given strategies for working through problems. Essentially, it works to help change the way you think (the cognitive part) and how you act (the behavioural part).

For example, if you are feeling fatigued and unable to achieve something you had set out to do today – like visiting a friend or finishing some work – this can, perhaps, lead to thoughts that you are useless and feelings of guilt. These, in turn, will bring down your mood, and this could change how you behave – say, by withdrawing even more. This creates a negative cycle, which CBT aims to help you recognise and break.

If you live in the UK, you can often access CBT through your family doctor, or you can self-refer. Another option is paying to see a private therapist (Resources, p. 359, has details for finding registered or accredited CBT therapists in the UK or Ireland), and some employers offer a limited number of free sessions to staff, so it is worth contacting your human-resources department about this.

There are also other talking treatments besides CBT. It is important to find the right person and psychological treatment to help you; it may be a psychologist, a psychotherapist or a counsellor. If your symptoms are also affecting your family or partner, then group or couple sessions may also be beneficial.

Exercise

Exercise can be a quick – and free – way to lift your mood and reinforce your self-worth. It often releases endorphins (so called feel-good chemicals) and expends any nervous energy you may be harbouring.[97]

If you feel like you need a pick-me-up right now, head to Chapter 10 for more exercise advice and inspiration. Many people find that regular exercise can be very mood-enhancing and beneficial.

Mindfulness

More and more of my patients are turning to mindfulness – the act of focusing on the present moment – as part of their mental-health first-aid kit. Studies have shown it can help with hot flushes and irritability.[98] You may be able to access some courses through your family doctor, or find a private teacher (see Resources, p. 357), and mindfulness is a practice that can also be carried out at home. Lots of my patients use meditation apps, and I've found the Headspace app (also in Resources) for mindfulness really useful in the past, alongside my regular yoga practice.

EXPERT VIEW
Mindfulness: finding calm in the midst of the menopause – Claudia Brown,
Yoga teacher with an interest in mindfulness

I've always been very vocal about how yoga and mindfulness have helped me through various times in my life, and especially during the perimenopause and menopause. But some people have remarked how they think this is a surprising admission from a medic like me.

Health and wellbeing aren't just about HRT; they go beyond that. You have to think holistically – and having a tool like mindfulness at your disposal can be incredibly useful when things feel overwhelming.

Claudia is a yoga teacher who has a passion for supporting women through their perimenopause and menopause, and we're so fortunate to have her expertise in running yoga workshops in my clinic and as a 'balance+ guru' for my app.

Over to Claudia . . .

Take a moment to think about when you were last on autopilot – that is, acting without stopping to think about what you are doing, usually because you have done it many times before. Perhaps it was while doing the supermarket shop at the weekend, or even having a shower this morning?

The importance of being versus doing

We lead such busy lives, trying to cram in as much as we can, so that we get caught up in multitasking and miss out on the messages our bodies are sending. When we are on autopilot, our minds are stuck in 'doing' mode: what we need to do is shift the focus from 'doing' to simply 'being' – fully present in the moment.

This is where mindfulness comes in.

Sometimes called embodied cognition, mindfulness is when you actively tune in to the messages your body is sending you. It's a form of meditation that focuses on thoughts, sensations and your surroundings, so that instead of feeling overwhelmed or ignoring them, you can acknowledge these thoughts and manage them.

How can mindfulness help you during the perimenopause and menopause?

Research shows that mindfulness helps with symptoms of stress, anxiety and other mental-health conditions, which may or may not be part of your menopause journey. Studies have shown that mindfulness has a positive impact on irritability, depression and anxiety in menopausal women.[99] Some studies also suggest it can help women manage the impact of hot flushes and night sweats.[100]

Getting started

One of the core tools of mindfulness practice is something called the body scan, which you can try at home.

The body scan takes about ten minutes and involves standing or sitting still with your eyes closed. Starting at the feet, direct your attention to each part of your body, noticing the sensations and feelings as you pass through – such as the sensation of a rug beneath your feet or the feeling of your chest rising and falling when you breathe in and out. Focus on each area of your body in turn, moving upwards before ending at the top of your head.

Another useful practice is mindful walking. Walking really lends itself to mindful practice, from the rhythm of putting one foot in front of the other, to noticing nature – the sights and sounds around you.

Where can I practise mindfulness?

In its truest form, mindfulness is a practice delivered by a qualified practitioner, often a mental-health professional or clinician. Practitioners in the UK tend to follow a format called mindfulness-based cognitive therapy (MBCT).

MBCT is usually a six- to eight-week course delivered in a group environment, with an emphasis on mindfulness practice every day during that period. Courses can include meditation, breathing exercises, mindful movement, body scanning, mindful eating, mindful walking and a variety of written work, which is integral to the structured programme.

Give yoga a try

One of the easiest ways to bring mindfulness into your life in a structured way is by doing a yoga class. While this is certainly not the same as an MBCT session (more often than not, a yoga teacher won't be a trained mental-health professional or a mindfulness practitioner), an experienced teacher will be able to introduce and guide you through mindful practices as part of the wider yoga experience.

In yoga, we teach a wide variety of breathing exercises, meditations and visualisations, moving the body in tune with the breath and mind. As an example, take the all-important savasana, the pose at the end of a yoga class where you lie down and take intentional rest: taking the time to rest and be in tune with your breath is the perfect opportunity to be mindful.

Mindfulness isn't a one-off

You need to practise mindfulness regularly to maintain the benefits it brings.

Think of it in the same way that you would physical exercise – if you don't work your muscles regularly, they lose strength.

And you don't need to be statue-still to practise mindfulness; you can do it when carrying out a gentle, repetitive hobby with a single pointed focus to quieten the mind, such as swimming, walking, knitting or even painting. Embrace slowing down and being in the moment.

My top three tips:

1. Stop: build time into your daily schedule to stop, breathe, move – and treat it as you would treat an important meeting.
2. Make an event of it: when you have decided what works for you (this could be a mindful shower or a mindful walk), really make an event of it and take in all five senses.

146

3. Be KIND to yourself: tame that inner critic, and remember –
    you can have awareness, but without compassion it isn't
    mindfulness.

Why antidepressants aren't usually a cure-all for perimenopause- and menopause-related low mood

The first time a woman comes to my clinic, they will be asked about their medical history and previous treatments they have taken or been recommended. The majority will have been offered and prescribed antidepressants to help with their moods.

Feeling down, sad and upset can be very common symptoms of the menopause and perimenopause. Other psychological symptoms include feelings of low self-esteem, reduced motivation or interest in things, anxiety and panic attacks, irritability and mood swings. It is clear to see why these feelings could be mistaken for depression and perhaps, therefore, understandable why a healthcare professional might prescribe antidepressants.

There is no evidence that antidepressants help to improve the psychological symptoms of the perimenopause and menopause. Yet, despite clear NICE guidelines, many women are still inappropriately offered anti-depressants when they first seek help from a healthcare professional for their menopausal symptoms.[101]

Clinical depression is a distinct mental-health condition for which antidepressants are a treatment. Antidepressants can be taken with HRT – in fact, studies have shown that they work better in the presence of oestradiol, so if you are offered them and you are perimenopausal or menopausal, you should also talk to your health-care professional about taking both.[102]

Studies have repeatedly shown that HRT containing oestrogen can improve depressive symptoms during the perimenopause and menopause.[103] Taking HRT during the perimenopause may also reduce the risk of depression occurring.[104] In addition, there is some evidence that psychosis due to schizophrenia can also improve with taking HRT.[105]

The right dose and type of HRT can often really improve these symptoms as this is treating the underlying cause. My clinical experience – and also that of other menopause experts – is that the addition of testosterone to oestrogen can be very beneficial to improve mood.

I am working with a team of menopause specialists and psych-iatrists (including the Royal College of Psychiatrists) to develop learn-ing programmes for healthcare professionals working in mental health to learn more about the importance of female hormones in our brains. We are also funding a PhD student who is specifically looking into the role of female hormones on suicide prevention and mental health.

CASE STUDY: MENTAL HEALTH, HRT AND ME – CLAIR'S STORY

Sometimes, changes to your mental health are one of the first signs of the perimenopause, particularly if you have struggled with PMS or anxiety and depression in the past. Clair shares her story here of how dips in her mental health before her periods worsened in her late thirties, and how – thanks to her knowledge as a GP – she knew her hormones might be to blame.

'I am in my early forties, and my mental health has always been a bit of a struggle at times. In my thirties, I began to notice quite a significant change in my symptoms around my menstrual cycle. I have been taking citalopram (an antidepressant) on and off for a number of years, to help control symptoms of anxiety and depression. As I approached forty, I began to find the PMS symptoms more and more difficult to control. I frequently felt suicidal in the lead-up to my period and would have intrusive thoughts that I found quite distressing.

'I am a GP and have a special interest in women's health, perimenopause and menopause. I have also learned a lot from my patients, so I tried to work out how best to manage my own symptoms. I took red clover, agnus castus, vitamin D, calcium and magnesium. I'd had CBT, and I tried to address factors in my lifestyle.

'I did see a little improvement but was still finding that in the lead-up to my periods, suicidal thoughts were commonplace. The next step was to try cycle suppression [using medication to stop your periods and avoid the resulting fluctuations in hormone levels].

'Although I have great faith in my GP, I wanted to discuss my options with a menopause specialist. I arranged an appointment at a private menopause clinic, explained my symptoms to the specialist and said that I wanted to try hormone replacement therapy (HRT). She was excellent, and agreed that HRT might help me. She prescribed Oestrogel and Utrogestan capsules and they have honestly been life-changing for me. They fit so nicely into my daily routine and were very easy to use.

'My symptoms began to improve very quickly; even in the first cycle, I noticed I felt much better in the lead-up to my period. The intrusive suicidal thoughts really eased, and I couldn't believe what a difference the HRT had made. Over the next few months, I increased my Oestrogel until I felt my symptoms were under as much control as they could be. I am now using four pumps of the gel and have also added testosterone, which has improved how I am feeling even further.

'My GP has been very supportive and took over prescribing the Oestrogel and Utrogestan, which was brilliant. I still continue to take citalopram, but I'm hoping I might be able to stop this and simply use the HRT to control my symptoms – the HRT has helped me more than the citalopram ever has.

'It is absolutely vital that the impact of perimenopause and menopause on our mental health is recognised. I was fortunate enough to realise that my changing hormones were what could have been making my symptoms worse, and I was able to access the right treatment. Had I not had this awareness and means to see a menopause specialist, who knows what the outcome may have been?'

I've been offered antidepressants, but I don't think I'm depressed. What now?

Be direct. Ask why you have been offered antidepressants, and in relation to which of your symptoms. The NICE guidelines state antidepressants should not be offered for low mood associated with the perimenopause or menopause, so ask your healthcare professional why they are being prescribed instead of HRT, the first-line treatment. You may need to see a different healthcare professional or ask to be referred to a menopause specialist.

Many women who are given antidepressants when they do

not have clinical depression explain that taking the antidepressants has made them feel numb, joyless and lacking in emotions (both happy and sad). Antidepressants also often cause reduced libido, and many women find they cannot orgasm when they are taking antidepressants. Some types of antidepressants have been shown to significantly increase fracture risk in perimenopausal women if taken for longer than five years.[106]

Having said all that, there may be circumstances where antidepressants can form part of a menopausal treatment plan. For example, in the case of a woman who is unable to take HRT or chooses not to, antidepressants can be offered to try to improve hot flushes, or for perimenopausal and menopausal women who also have clinical depression.

Timeout #1: Unwind in five steps

1. 'Check in': try to check in with yourself during the day to pinpoint how you are feeling and prevent a build-up of tension, asking yourself:
    - Do I need to relax my shoulders?
    - Do I need to take some deep breaths?
    - Do I need to try to clear my mind for a few moments?
2. Plan ahead: if you have a stressful event on the horizon, tackle it head on by making a to-do list and splitting up bigger jobs into smaller tasks to make the situation feel more manageable.

3. **Positive thoughts:** if you are experiencing a crisis of confidence, consider what your best friend would say to support you if they were in front of you right now.

4. **The power of reflection:** take a few minutes towards the end of each day to reflect on what went well, what you have achieved and what you are grateful for.

5. **Be active:** if you are feeling restless, channel that energy into an activity to lift your spirits and expend it, be it a short walk or a full-blown exercise class.

Menopause and coping with other mental-health conditions

You may be heading into – or already experiencing – menopausal symptoms while coping with another mental-health condition. In fact, about one in five women in England alone has a common mental-health problem such as depression and anxiety, so you would be in good company.

At the moment, little research exists into the relationship between hormones and other mental-health conditions, including serious lifelong mood disorders. But what we do know is that women who have a prior history of PMS, PMDD or postnatal depression (see pp. 14–30) after giving birth are more likely to suffer from low mood in menopause. We also know that women with attention deficit hyperactivity disorder are more likely to suffer from PMDD, and women with biopolar are most sensitive to hormonal shifts during the perimenopause and menopause.[107]

But clearly, much more research is needed to ensure all women receive truly holistic care.

Having an existing mental-health condition and being menopausal can be challenging on a number of fronts. Firstly, if you start to experience low-mood symptoms, it can be difficult to know which are down to your existing mental-health condition and which are new and hormone-related. Secondly, your existing healthcare team may assume these new symptoms are part of your diagnosis without exploring further – in medicine this is known as diagnostic overshadowing.

So how can you help yourself?

You can start by tracking to record any new symptoms that you think are menopause-related, so you can build up as full a picture as possible before making an appointment with a healthcare professional (this may be your family doctor or a mental health specialist). Then, when you book the appointment, make it clear that you wish to discuss the menopause, and take with you any notes you have made. You may also want to take a friend or relative with you if you feel you would benefit from their support.

It is really important not to stop taking any current medication or halt any agreed treatment plans without consulting your healthcare professional. The goal, if you are perimenopausal or menopausal, should be to carry on treating your existing condition, while tackling menopause symptoms at the same time.

CASE STUDY: HORMONE CHANGES
AND OBSESSIVE-COMPULSIVE
DISORDER – ANNA'S STORY

Anna had a history of OCD and bouts of depression, but her mental health had been stable for twelve years. Then, at the age of forty-five, she fell into a deep depression that left her suicidal.

'I had severe postnatal depression (PND) after the birth of my first child but I had been stable and happy on a medium dose of antidepressants. I wouldn't say my OCD was cured, but it was very low-level indeed, and wasn't interfering with my day-to-day life.

'Then, last year, I was hit out of the blue with a sudden deterioration in my OCD with no apparent cause. Given my serious history, as soon as I realised I was feeling very low and my OCD had flared up, I asked for an immediate referral to a private psychiatrist. He said my symptoms were most likely due to stress, as I'd recently been ill with COVID-19 and had also been through a court battle with the council to get specialist education for my daughter. So he increased my antidepressant dosage – but it didn't help.

'I began to spiral until, eventually, I was suicidal and on two high-dose antidepressants, an antipsychotic, tranquillisers and sleeping pills. I was hospitalised, and I gradually improved and was taken off the tranquillisers and sleeping pills. Although the deep depression had lifted, I still felt very flat and anxious – which I never had before. I couldn't remember what it felt like to be happy or excited about anything.

'In the hospital I had terrible night sweats, and would wake up soaking wet, but I assumed it was a side effect of all the medications. I was often setting the air-con to 17°, and the nurses would come in every morning and tell me that the room was absolutely freezing. But at first, no one connected the dots, myself included. I

154

honestly thought that I didn't need to be aware of the menopause until my late fifties or early sixties, and I had no idea that forty-five is actually a fairly average age to be starting the perimenopause.

'When I finally began to suspect that perimenopause could be a factor, I contacted my psychiatrist (who has many decades of experience) on two occasions to ask him if he thought it could be relevant. I was hoping he would want to be involved in treating my perimenopausal symptoms because I was already on so many drugs – and I didn't really want someone new involved in my care. Unfortunately, this didn't happen, so I sought help via a menopause specialist.

'When I started taking HRT, I felt better almost straight away. The only way to describe it is like my brain had been turned off and someone had just switched it back on. I can't say for sure that my symptoms were caused by hormonal changes. All I know is that I've improved hugely since being on HRT – but I'm also still on the two antidepressants and an antipsychotic, so it's possible that it's a combination of everything that's made me feel better. My husband is convinced that my symptoms were linked to hormones – I was doing a lot of crying, but he says his shoulders have finally dried off!

'I desperately wish I had known that previous mental-health difficulties, especially PMS and PND, would make me more susceptible to mental-health issues during the menopause. Of course, not all women who have had PND will struggle, but I think it's important to be aware and informed, as I could have been much better prepared.

'On a practical note, I'd recommend that any woman who is suffering from mental-health issues should talk to their doctor and persist if they don't get appropriate help at first. No woman aged forty-five should sit in a psychiatric hospital for four weeks without hormones being mentioned once. I think menopause needs to be kept in mind as a possible factor in mental illness in women of any age, but particularly in those over thirty-five. It makes me incredibly sad to think that if only the first psychiatrist I saw had tried me on HRT, as well as increasing my antidepressants, then my family and I could have been saved from so much pain and suffering.'

How do you sleep at night?

In these busy times, we can often look upon getting a good night's sleep as a luxury, rather than what it is: an essential contributor to a healthy functioning brain and body.

I'm very protective of my sleep. I like to go to bed and get up at the same times every day to establish a routine, even at the weekends. I try to close my laptop and other electronic devices at a sensible hour, so I can wind down before my head hits the pillow. Of course, there will be the odd late night or family holiday that means I don't always keep to the routine, but I do my best to stick to it. I also know that altered routines can trigger migraines, too.

So before we end this chapter with Dr David Garley's explainer on the link between mental health and sleep, let's take a few minutes to think about your sleep over the past few nights:

- What time have you been getting to bed?
- Do you always go to bed and get up at the same time?
- What have you eaten for your evening meals – a light supper or heavy meal? Any alcohol?
- What time did you eat?

- What is your bedtime routine? A long bath and a book in bed, or do you fall asleep on the sofa most nights?
- How do you create a calm atmosphere in your bedroom?
- Do you need to switch that phone off?

EXPERT VIEW

How sleep affects your mental health in menopause – Dr David Garley,

Managing Director of the Better Sleep Clinic, Bristol

As a 'balance+ guru', Dr David is the expert on all things sleep-related. He worked in an NHS sleep clinic before moving into general practice and opening The Better Sleep Clinic.

Low mood and anxiety can be common features of the perimenopause and menopause due to the fluctuating and falling hormones, but changes to your sleep can also have a real impact on your mental health.

Unfortunately, the amount and quality of your sleep can be affected during this time; this could be due to night-time waking because of sweats, or simply having the urge to go to the toilet more because of urinary symptoms. The menopause could also coincide with the development of a sleeping disorder like sleep apnoea, where your breathing repeatedly stops and starts while you sleep.

Read on to learn how poor sleep affects your mental health:

Low mood and depression

It is well established that depression leads to poor-quality sleep, and this frequently manifests as early-morning waking. However, it is becoming increasingly understood that poor sleep can be a trigger for depression, as well as a by-product.

This perhaps isn't so surprising when you think about how you feel after a terrible night's sleep – terms like edgy, irritable and emotional come to mind. If your sleep is consistently poor night after night, then features of depression – such as low mood, lack of motivation and a lack of enjoyment in life – may present themselves.

Anxiety

Anxiety is a common reason why patients say they have trouble falling asleep; your mind may be racing or you are experiencing worrying thoughts that refuse to go away. You might find yourself waking in the middle of the night and ruminating over things you said (or didn't say) and this stops you getting back to sleep. As with low mood, sleep and anxiety have a similar two-way causality.

Rapid eye movement (REM) sleep

Part of this two-way relationship between your sleep and mental health is down to the functions that good sleep provides, particularly the REM stage of sleep.

REM sleep is the stage where your most vivid dreams occur. It is also where you process the emotional thoughts and experiences from the day, which leads to better regulation of emotions the following day.

Most of your REM sleep occurs towards the end of the night, during the few hours before you get up. Studies have shown that the onset of depression can be preceded by reduced REM sleep.[108]

Ways to improve your sleep and mental health

When mental-health conditions are both a cause and effect of poor sleep, it tends to fuel the process and become a vicious cycle, with one problem feeding the other. It is important to break this cycle by tackling your mental health and your sleep at the same time.

- Hormones: if you are struggling with multiple menopausal symptoms, consider taking HRT to top up or replace your missing hormones and give your sleep and mental health the best chance to improve.
- Practise good sleep hygiene: try to go to bed and get up at the same times every day, avoid heavy meals that take a long time to digest too close to bedtime and don't immediately reach for your phone on the bedside table when you can't sleep.
- Prioritise self-care: eat a balanced diet, exercise regularly and talk about how you are feeling with friends and family.
- See a healthcare professional for specific sleep disorders (like sleep apnoea or insomnia): it's important that these are diagnosed and treated effectively.

And if your sleep still doesn't improve with these measures, speak to a healthcare professional, so they can help direct you to more focused treatments.

SURVEY: MENOPAUSE AND MENTAL HEALTH

An overwhelming 95 per cent of respondents to my survey said they had experienced a negative change in their mood and emotions since becoming perimenopausal or menopausal.

The most commonly reported symptoms were stress and anxiety, followed by feeling more easily overwhelmed, feeling low or tearful and feeling angry or irritable. Of those who sought help from a healthcare professional about their perimenopause or menopause symptoms, more than a third (38 per cent) said they were offered antidepressants instead of HRT.

6

Skin and Hair in the Menopause

Four things you will learn in this chapter:

1. How hormones support healthy skin and hair

2. Hair and skin changes that can occur during the perimenopause and menopause

3. Do I need a menopause moisturiser? Building a skincare routine to suit you

4. All about caring for your hair

Until recently, menopause was a word barely mentioned in the £5.5-billion-a-year UK health-and-beauty industry.[109] For decades, the focus for mid-life skin and hair was on 'mature', dry skin, 'dry, damaged' hair or anti-ageing formulas. But there is now a burgeoning market of products promising to tackle menopause-related skincare and hair concerns.

This chapter really focuses on the science of how the menopause affects skin, looking at the common conditions that can occur and, most importantly, how to tackle them, as well as giving you some practical tips that you can start trying today. Lending his considerable expertise is Dr Sajjad Rajpar, a consultant dermatologist who has a special interest in skin and hair changes during the perimenopause and menopause. He's a regular expert on my balance app and is going to be giving you some solid advice on how to develop a skincare routine to help you.

But it's not just about skin – I will be looking at hair, too, which can really impact on your self-esteem. I will also be concentrating on areas such as female-pattern hair loss and excess facial hair, with some practical suggestions on how to tackle both and on how to care for your hair in general.

Skin- and haircare can be confusing – and often expensive. Who hasn't bought the latest lotion or potion in the hope that their skin and hair concerns will be resolved overnight? But before you go rushing out and blowing your budget on a whole new regime (or start borrowing your teen's spot cream), read on.

What's happening to my skin?

Dry, parched, sallow and even spotty? If you are experiencing skin changes during the perimenopause and menopause, believe me, you are not the only one.

A few years ago, I remember staring in the mirror while getting ready for an evening out with friends. I'd been rushing around all day – seeing patients, school runs and general life admin – and it was probably the first time in a long while that I'd taken a

THE DEFINITIVE GUIDE TO THE PERIMENOPAUSE AND MENOPAUSE

few minutes to look at my face. Not just a cursory look while I was my brushing my teeth, but I mean *really* staring hard into the mirror.

Performing what can only be described as facial gymnastics, I started pressing my hands to my face, examining the laughter lines around my eyes and frown lines on my forehead. As I tilted my head this way and that, I found lines I'd never noticed before, my skin felt looser with less tone and I felt thoroughly fed up.

In short, when I hit the perimenopause, my skin changed. The tried-and-tested products that had been a staple of my bathroom cabinet throughout my thirties and early forties just didn't seem to be cutting the mustard any longer. My complexion felt sallow, lifeless and, at times, a bit sore. If I had a bad night's sleep – which, thanks to night sweats and low hormone levels, was a pretty common occurrence – it showed in my face the next morning. Whereas before, a little make-up covered up the signs of fatigue and gave me a bit of a glow, now it just didn't sit on my skin that well.

As my reflection stared back at me, I felt pretty deflated. I'd been reasonably healthy all my life: I'd never smoked, always ate healthily, guzzled water and had tried to look after my skin. What could I do to fix it?

My first thought was that I needed to get moisture back into my face, so I bought a super-rich night cream and slathered it on my face every night in the hope it would give my skin a boost. But instead of making my parched face feel hydrated and comforted, I was left with greasy skin and spots around my nose and along my hairline.

For me, the perimenopause showed in my skin with dryness,

fine lines and dullness, but for others it can see the return of teenage acne or pigmentation. One survey shows that 46 per cent of women attending a menopause clinic had skin issues arising from the menopause.[110]

As the largest organ of your body, your skin can suffer from the lack of oestrogen during perimenopause and menopause. Oestrogen is required for your skin's natural hydration mechanisms because it helps your skin produce four key substances:

- **Ceramides:** oils (known as lipids) that help to maintain the integrity of your skin's barrier and keep out irritants
- **Natural hyaluronic acid:** sitting just below your skin's surface, hyaluronic acid helps your skin to retain water
- **Sebum:** produced in the sebaceous glands, this is an oily substance that forms a protective barrier to help protect and moisturise your skin; too little, and your skin becomes dry; too much, and your skin becomes oily and can clog the pores, leading to spots
- **Collagen:** a supporting protein that provides structure to your skin

Hormones and your skin

As oestrogen levels reduce during the perimenopause and menopause, your skin can become thinner and less supple. The low oestrogen levels can result in there being less blood flowing to the epidermis (upper layer of your skin) and more water loss from your skin, leading to your skin being less hydrated.[111] As you age, the skin also loses elastin, another protein, which provides stretchiness in your body.

Testosterone is also likely to have a beneficial effect on skin and hair – we hear many women tell us that their skin feels and looks better and their hair grows quicker and thicker when they are using testosterone.

CASE STUDY: COPING WITH ACNE AND THE MENOPAUSE – ANGELA'S STORY

Angela has suffered with cystic acne (a severe and painful form of the condition, where pus-filled acne cysts form deep under the skin) since she was a teenager.

Here she talks about her year-long journey to reach a menopause diagnosis, and the challenges of coping with the menopause and a pre-existing skin condition.

'My symptoms started about ten years ago, when I was forty-five. I started experiencing numerous unexplained symptoms like bad anxiety, palpitations and memory trouble.

'I first developed cystic acne when I was eighteen, and, while the acne itself didn't get any worse, at the same time I was getting all these new symptoms, my skin changed, too: up until my mid-forties I was dealing with cystic acne and oily skin, but now my skin felt very dry and tight.

'I went to my GP and was sent off on a whirlwind of appointments – cardiology for the palpitations, a memory clinic and MRI scans for the forgetfulness. It was a really scary time: I wasn't getting any answers and it was hard not to focus on the prospect of Alzheimer's disease, heart problems or even an early death.

'After a year of various investigations, I was still no closer to a diagnosis. I'm a nurse practitioner, so I put my professional hat on and went away and did some research myself, and menopause came back as the common denominator for pretty much all the symptoms I'd been experiencing.

'I took this back to my GP and said, "I know we've been looking at these different tests, but do you think it could be the perimenopause?"

'He agreed and referred me to a really great local menopause clinic. I saw a menopause specialist, was prescribed HRT and, within weeks, I was back to my normal self. It was a huge relief after all those months of worry.

'That was ten years ago, and I haven't needed to go back to the clinic since. I'm under the care of my local GP and still take HRT, but have adjusted it a few times, based on availability of different preparations and the latest research.

'I've also transformed my lifestyle in the last decade; I've given up alcohol, eat a balanced diet and I'm addicted to yoga and Pilates.

'Unfortunately, my cystic acne hasn't cleared up, and all the mask-wearing at work during the pandemic definitely didn't help, so it's really a question of trying to keep it under control. Cystic acne and drier skin – it's a real balancing act. I take antibiotics to help reduce bacteria and inflammation and concentrate on products that keep the moisture in.

'But when I look back on my life now compared to ten years ago, I'm in a much better place. I'm more active, healthier and in control of my hormones.'

Common skin problems during perimenopause and menopause

Let's look at some of the most widespread skin conditions that can occur during the perimenopause and menopause, and some simple suggestions on how to tackle them.

Itching and dry skin

The most common complaint from women I treat around the time of the menopause is itching and dry skin. Without the right levels of ceramides, hyaluronic acid, sebum and collagen, water evaporates very easily, causing the skin to become dry and scaly.

What you can do

HRT will help to replace the lost oestrogen and you should start to see an improvement in the feel and texture of your skin within a few months.

However, there are many other steps you can take – and products you should avoid – to improve things.

Soap can be very drying on your face and body, so it is best to avoid products that lather, foam or bubble, as these will simply strip away grease from your skin.

Use a gentle non-foaming cleanser on your body instead of soap. And if you suffer from dry skin on your hands, use a moisturising lotion as a cleanser in place of hand soap when washing them.

Use a facial moisturiser twice a day – a lighter one in the daytime and something heavier at night. Try to get into the habit of moisturising your skin immediately after a shower or bath, as this helps your skin to hold on to more water and can prevent it from drying out.

There are other causes of itching, aside from dry skin. Sometimes it can be related to release of histamine in your skin and irritation of skin nerves can give the sensation of insects creeping on your skin (known as formication). Other causes of itching are iron deficiency and thyroid disturbance. It may be worth reviewing these possible causes with a healthcare professional.

Redness and flushing

Flushing is a well-recognised symptom of the menopause. It can also occur with rosacea, a condition in which your blood vessels in the skin become very reactive. Rosacea appears to be more common in women, especially during the menopause.

What you can do

Redness and flushing from rosacea can often improve with simple lifestyle changes, such as cutting down your intake of alcohol and caffeine, avoiding spicy foods and protecting your skin from the sun. Sometimes additional measures may be required, such as creams or laser treatments that help to shrink tiny blood vessels in your skin. Speak to a healthcare professional about options that may be suitable for you.

Spots and other types of acne

Spots can be very distressing at any stage in life, but particularly when they occur around the menopause. Many women – especially those who had acne as teenagers – have flare-ups around the menopause and it is not clear why. It's possible that a drop in oestrogen means the ratio of male hormones is relatively higher, and this may trigger the condition. For some, acne continues to be a problem, even following oestrogen replacement.

What you can do

Take a good look through your make-up and sun-protection products and check that they are all suitable for oily or combination skins, or described as 'non-comedogenic' (this means they are not going to clog your pores and aggravate acne). Also check the expiry dates, as most sunscreens should only be used for twelve months after opening. Use a mild cleanser that contains salicylic acid, as this will help to exfoliate your skin and unblock pores. Active ingredients like retinol and niacinamide are useful to include in a skincare regime if you are prone to outbreaks. And remember, it can take a couple of months for skin products to work for acne, so be patient.

Timeout #1: Look at your skin

Spend a few minutes looking in the mirror at your skin:

- Has the texture changed in recent weeks or months?
- Are there any new marks, moles or spots you are concerned about?
- Are the changes causing discomfort, pain or embarrassment?
- How would you describe the look and feel of your skin in five words?

Sun damage

Signs of sun damage may become more prominent around the menopause, especially for anyone who has spent a considerable amount of time in the sun over their lifetime.[112] Signs of sun damage can include irregular skin tone, lacklustre skin and sun spots (flat brown marks that show up on your face, décolleté and arms – also known as age spots). Thread veins, lines or wrinkles may also develop.

What you can do

Avoid tanning and any skin burning by wearing a sunscreen with a high sun-protection factor (SPF), such as factor 50. Remember to reapply sunscreen every two hours when you are out in the sun. Also, wear long sleeves and a hat with a wide brim where possible. If you are worried about any dark sun spots or changing moles, see a healthcare professional.

Bruising, fragile skin and slow wound healing

Your skin can become thinner and more fragile as you get older, and a lack of oestrogen can exacerbate this process due to the slowing down of collagen production, meaning that skin can become weaker.[113]

Bruising is also caused by a reduction in collagen around the tiny blood vessels in your skin. With a lack of collagen, even the slightest knock can produce a bruise. Wounds also take longer to heal in those with low oestrogen levels.

What you can do

Consider replacing your lost oestrogen by taking HRT, sooner rather than later, as this can help to preserve your skin's collagen levels.

Wrinkles, jowls and dull skin

The change in facial appearance that occurs with the menopause can be very distressing for many and can severely affect self-confidence and quality of life. I know it certainly did for me.

Research shows that during the menopause, women lose bone density (bone strength) from the facial bones – as well as elsewhere in the body – and that this may contribute to many of the facial changes they notice.[114] Bones can become smaller (as old bone tissue is lost faster than new bone tissue grows – see p. 97), and in the spine and limbs this loss of bone tissue and strength makes women more prone to fractures. On your face, the loss in bone mass can cause hollowing in the mid face, narrowing of the chin, jowls and loss of jawline definition.

The drop in collagen means skin can lose its tightness and become more prone to fine lines and wrinkles, which add to the signs of ageing. An estimated 30 per cent of skin collagen may be lost in the first five years after the menopause.[115]

What you can do

The most important changes you can make are to cut out habits that cause skin collagen levels to decline, such as damaging sun exposure and smoking. Once these issues are addressed, serums that contain anti-ageing ingredients to help preserve skin collagen levels (including topical retinoids and vitamin C) can be helpful.

EXPERT VIEW
How to develop a skincare routine that works for you – Dr Sajjad Rajpar,
Consultant Dermatologist

Dr Sajjad has been a consultant dermatologist for over a decade. He's brilliant at debunking skincare myths and looking beyond the fancy packaging of various lotions and potions, to get to the science to help *you* establish simple but effective skincare routines.

I've spent more than a decade helping women with skin concerns related to their perimenopause and menopause.

Women will often ask me for advice on the changes they can make during the perimenopause and menopause and for me, there are two key things: firstly, always speak to a professional if anything about your skin is bothering you; and secondly, try to establish some consistency with your skin with a good skincare routine.

We often hear the term 'skincare routine' but what does that actually mean?

A skincare routine is about using products regularly to maintain healthy skin; to treat concerns such as dryness and to prevent others such as signs of ageing, you need to be consistent. And because everyone's menopause is different, and that is particularly true when it comes to taking care of skin, the routine needs to be unique to your needs and concerns. What works for someone with greasy skin and breakouts won't work for you if you are suffering from dry, itchy skin.

In addition, a routine needn't be complicated. You don't need dozens of products or have to switch every few weeks. Nor does it have to be pricy; there are lots of excellent products out there and you shouldn't feel you have to buy one brand's entire line of skincare.

So what does a good routine look like? There are four components:

- Cleanser
- Moisturiser
- Actives
- Sunscreen

Cleanser

This will remove dirt from the environment that has built up on your skin, grease, bacteria and dead skin cells that are ready to shed. Ideally, you'll want to cleanse twice a day – first thing in the morning and again in the evening.

The type of cleanser you use depends on your skin. If your skin is sensitive, you should go for something gentle and preferably non-foaming. If your skin is a bit more resilient or greasy and doesn't get too irritated, then you should be able to tolerate a stronger cleanser.

Moisturiser

This helps to keep the skin hydrated and supple and reduces itching. This is really important during the perimenopause and menopause as, without oestrogen, your skin's natural hydrating mechanisms have been compromised – so adding in moisturisers will improve the quality and health of your skin.

Light moisturisers are easily absorbed and heavier ones tend to be more ointment based. The general rule of thumb is that the drier your skin, the heavier the moisturiser should be. But remember that if you use a very heavy moisturiser, you could then be prone to outbreaks of acne – so if you have a history of acne, you might want to try something lighter.

Actives

Actives refers to products that change the biology of the skin. Your doctor might prescribe an active cream, or you might buy something over the counter to reduce skin ageing, control breakouts or control pigmentation or rosacea.

Examples of actives that might be used in a skincare regime include:

- retinols, which reduce skin ageing and help boost collagen
- niacinamide, which reduces pigmentation and can also help with breakouts and redness
- peptides, which can stimulate collagen production
- vitamin C, an antioxidant that can help reduce skin ageing
- ferulic acid, another antioxidant that reduces skin ageing.

Sunscreen

A sunscreen blocks UVA and UVB – wavelengths of light that can cause skin cancer and skin ageing. Sunscreen is particularly important during the perimenopause and menopause because, without oestrogen, your skin is likely to age at a much faster rate.

Do you need a dedicated menopause moisturiser or other products?

There has been a rise in menopause-branded hair and skincare products in recent years, but many non-specialised ones can help with perimenopausal and menopausal skincare concerns, alongside HRT. For example, active ingredients that change the biology of the skin, such as retinols or niacinamide, can be found in numerous products – even some marketed at men.

My advice is that you look at a product's ingredients, rather than the branding, and that you study your skin to establish

173

what you really need (not what you think you might need); your skincare routine should be unique to you.

Putting the four skincare-regime components into practice
No one size fits all when it comes to a skincare routine, but here are some guidelines.

If you have very resilient skin and want to tackle ageing, you could try the following:

Morning:
- Non-foaming hydrating cleanser, followed by an active product, such as vitamin C or a combination product containing vitamin C or ferulic acid
- Moisturiser
- Sunscreen, if going out

Evening:
- Micellar water – a solution made up of purified water, moisturiser and cleanser, to remove make-up, followed by a second hydrating cleanser
- Moisturiser
- Retinoid

If your skin is very dry or sensitive, then the above routine would be too harsh. Instead, you could try the following:

Morning:
- Moisturising wash
- Moisturiser
- Sunscreen

Evening:

- Repeat the same routine, minus the sunscreen.

Remember: try to be patient, as it can take some time – even a few months – for changes to be seen. And it's important not to change your entire routine in one day; only change one product at a time, so you can see how your skin reacts.

Hair changes during the perimenopause and menopause

Long, short, curly or straight, hair is such an incredibly important part of our self-image. For some of us, our hair is a form of armour, while bolder styles may be an expression of our personalities. So when hair changes start creeping in during perimenopause and menopause, it can have a devastating impact on self-esteem.

I will freely admit, I am pretty useless when it comes to styling my hair (just ask my daughters), so I've come to love a simple bob that is easy to style. And I've been quite fortunate in that my hair didn't suffer too much during the early days of perimenopause before I started taking HRT.

I've been going to my hairdresser, Matthew Curtis, for several years now, and he has become something of a confidant. It's probably no surprise that one of the main topics we chat about during appointments is the menopause and hair, because, like me, Matthew sees the impact of hair loss or other challenges on women. It's something we both feel passionately should be talked about more – and more openly. So much so that when one of my regular hair appointments was cancelled due to COVID restrictions we decided to hop online instead and have a live IG chat about the impact of hormones on our hair!

So let's take a look at some of the common hair issues during the menopause – why they happen and what you can do about them.

Timeout #2: Look at your hair

Spend a few minutes looking at your hair:

- Do you notice any thinning in particular areas?
- How often are you using heated styling products – and for how long?
- Take a look at your comb or the bristles on your hairbrush – are any broken? Could they do with being replaced?

Hair loss

About 40 per cent of women will experience hair loss during or after menopause, in part because of the deficiency of hormones. Many of the cells in your skin and hair roots contain oestrogen receptors, so oestrogen directly stimulates these cells and these hairs.[116] Without it, your hair doesn't grow as strong or as thick.

Can HRT help with hair loss?

Unfortunately, there aren't enough studies to definitively state what proportion of women benefit from HRT in terms of hair loss. However, anecdotally, many patients notice their hair feels stronger and thicker after starting HRT.

But for some women, HRT may not improve hair loss. This is probably because it is down to other reasons, such as hereditary factors, stress, nutrition deficiency or immune disorders.[117]

Facial-hair growth

Some women notice they have thick hairs developing on the upper lip, chin, cheeks and jawline during perimenopause/ menopause. These can be related to a hormone imbalance or can occur for other reasons.

What you can do

This can be a distressing issue and there are several options to try. Hair-removal methods include plucking, waxing, threading, shaving and depilatory creams. Electrolysis and laser hair removal can offer a more permanent solution to unwanted hair. A prescription cream is also available to help slow down the rate of hair growth.

EXPERT VIEW
How to care for your hair during the perimenopause and menopause – Dr Sajjad Rajpar,
Consultant Dermatologist

- Be gentle: use a high-quality brush and avoid prolonged, high heat. Heat damages the hair by altering the keratin, which leads to reduced elasticity and strength, thinning and shedding.
- Hair roots don't like traction on them, so avoid tight hairstyles that can pull on them and exacerbate hair loss. For the same reason, avoid extensions as they could put weight on your hair.
- Don't over-colour the hair, as this can damage the hair shafts.

- Eat a balanced diet and, if you are planning on losing weight, do it gradually – crash diets can lead to hair loss.
- Speak to a healthcare professional – you might want to see your family doctor or a dermatologist who specialises in hair loss to establish a diagnosis to improve the hair or slow the rate of hair loss.
- Don't forget mental-health support; hair loss, in particular, can be devastating – so get support from family, friends or mental-health professionals.
- Look at cosmetic improvements – speak to your hairdresser about a volume-enhancing style, wigs or hair pieces. Another option is using a root spray (a coloured spray applied to the roots to conceal thinning areas).

SURVEY: SKIN DEEP – LOOKING AT THE IMPACT ON HAIR AND SKIN

Survey findings lay bare how skin and hair changes are a real source of worry for some.

Almost two thirds (64 per cent) of survey respondents said they had experienced dry skin, 56 per cent had itchy skin and 30 per cent said they had developed spots and/or acne.

Interestingly, 22 per cent reported a crawling sensation known as formication.

These symptoms also had an impact on skincare routines and skincare spending habits with a rise in spending.

When it came to hair, respondents reported symptoms including dryness, thinning and hair breakage, while 11 per cent said they had purchased specific menopause haircare products in the past 12 months.

7

Menopause in Younger People (Including Surgical Menopause)

Four things you will learn in this chapter:

1. What are early menopause and premature ovarian insufficiency (POI)?

2. What is surgical menopause?

3. Why your diagnosis journey may differ from an older woman's

4. The long-term health risks of an earlier menopause and a surgical menopause – and the treatments that can safeguard and improve your future health

We've all seen the pictures in magazines and on websites. Mostly, when the word menopause is used in the media, it'll be accompanied by a middle-aged, usually White female fanning herself on a hot day, frowning and making a 'wow-it's-really-hot-in-here'-type face.

If you went by pictures alone, you'd think the menopause only happened to women past the age of fifty, and hot flushes were the only symptom. And if you did, you couldn't be more wrong on both counts.

I was pretty much Ms Average when it came to my own peri-menopause. I first experienced symptoms in my mid-forties (a very common age to be perimenopausal) and started taking HRT not long after. As I am taking HRT, I will never know when I will be officially menopausal (I would have to stop it for one year and wait to see if I have a period in that time or not; I am certainly not going to do this!).

The perimenopause and menopause can be far from predict-able. For some women, it can happen years – even decades – before they expect it to. The youngest patient I have personally treated only had one natural period and became menopausal aged twelve.

When we talk about an 'early menopause', we are referring to menopause before the age of forty-five. And in women under forty, it is known as premature ovarian insufficiency (POI). Perhaps you are reading this chapter because you are in your thirties, twenties or even teens and suspect you may be display-ing the signs and symptoms of an earlier menopause and are looking for some guidance on what to do next? Or maybe you are supporting a friend or family member? Going through the menopause at an earlier age throws up different challenges – the absolute shock of the diagnosis, issues around fertility and the long-term health risks of depleted oestrogen compared to other women of your age. But one thing is for certain: you can start finding answers here in helping you to reach a diagnosis, come to terms with it and treat it.

What is an early menopause?

As we have covered, the average age of menopause is fifty-one. If you go through menopause between the ages of forty and forty-five, it is known as an early menopause; this affects approximately 5 per cent of the female population.[118]

The range of symptoms you can experience during an early menopause is the same as menopause at a 'normal' age. But if you aren't expecting it, it is easy for these to go under the radar or be incorrectly blamed on another condition entirely.

I've treated several women in their early forties who have been referred to specialists for all manner of tests before the penny has dropped that the root cause is the menopause. I've known patients who have had brain scans because of memory slips, and others who have been asked to wear a heart monitor to get to the bottom of their palpitations.

So being aware that menopause can happen earlier is being prepared. I'd recommend women of all ages who are having periods to use a tracker (such as the one on the balance app) to track flow and frequency, as well as symptoms and irregularities for discussion with a healthcare professional.

What is premature ovarian insufficiency (POI)?

POI is when menopause occurs before the age of forty and your ovaries no longer function as they should. It's actually more common than you might think. Approximately 1 in every 100 women under the age of 40, 1 in 1,000 women under 30 and 1 in 10,000 under 20 experience POI.

In both POI and early menopause, your ovaries no longer produce adequate amounts of hormones, including oestrogen and testosterone. This means that periods usually stop altogether, and you may experience symptoms of the menopause. Many women with POI and early menopause will have been perimenopausal before their periods stop – so they will have been experiencing menopausal symptoms and irregular (or even regular) periods for months or even years.

However, in many cases of POI your ovaries often do not completely fail, which is different to the natural menopause in middle age. This means that the function of your ovaries can fluctuate over time, occasionally resulting in a period, ovulation or even pregnancy, sometimes several years after diagnosis. This intermittent temporary return of ovarian function can result in around 5–10 per cent of women with POI being able to conceive.[119]

What causes POI and early menopause?

For most women with POI and early menopause, we just don't know what the underlying cause is. This is known in medical terms as 'idiopathic'. There are, however, some known causes.

The first is 'iatrogenic', meaning it is a result of medical treatment. I know that sounds strange – why on earth would you want to force the menopause on someone younger? But it can, in fact, be a side effect of some drugs or surgeries used to treat disease or another medical condition. Many drugs (such as aromatase inhibitors, given to some women who have had breast cancer) reduce the amount of oestrogen in your body and can lead to an early menopause. It can also be a result of having your ovaries surgically removed due to conditions like cysts or endometriosis. It can also be caused by radiotherapy to your pelvic area as a treatment for cancer, or certain types of chemotherapy drugs (used, for example, in women who had childhood cancer, or in their twenties or thirties). This loss of ovarian function can be temporary or permanent.

If both of your ovaries are surgically removed, this will result in you becoming menopausal straight away, as the ovaries will no longer produce any hormones. Some specialists refer to this as a bilateral oophorectomy without using the word menopause. Others refer to it as a surgical menopause. Having your womb removed during a hysterectomy can also result in an early menopause or POI, even if your ovaries are not removed.

Although your ovaries may still make some oestrogen and testosterone after a hysterectomy, it is likely your hormone levels will fall at an earlier age than average. We know from studies that a third to a half of women will have an earlier menopause after a hysterectomy, even though their ovaries are intact.[120] We're not entirely sure why, but one theory is that it is because the blood supply to your ovaries is affected by your uterus being removed.

In addition, women who have autoimmune diseases (where the body attacks its own cells) are more likely to have POI – for example, Addison's disease, thyroid disease, diabetes and coeliac disease are all autoimmune diseases.

Genetic conditions such as fragile X syndrome and Turner syndrome may also lead to POI, but this is very rare and, if it does occur, it is more likely in much younger women.

You may also find that a female relative like your mother,

grandmother, sister, aunt or cousin had an earlier menopause, so it is always worth asking the question among female members of your family. Although POI is not usually inherited, menopause at a young age can often run in families.

As explained, the symptoms of the perimenopause and menopause in younger women are the same as those experienced by older women. However, some women with POI or early menopause do not experience any or many symptoms. Hormone levels will be low regardless of whether or not symptoms occur.

CASE STUDY: POI DIAGNOSIS AT AGE FOURTEEN – ELLIE'S STORY

When Ellie Waters was fourteen years old, she was diagnosed with a soft-tissue cancer that required intensive and lengthy treatment. The interventions saved her life, but they also meant she became menopausal.

Ellie is an incredible, intelligent and articulate young woman. I was fortunate to have her as a guest on my podcast, and she also helped me to create resources especially for younger women going through the menopause you can follow her on Instagram @teamellie_blog.

'My story begins with just a small lump in my buttock that I thought would go away – even though it was clearly getting bigger. I then began having pain in my leg and severe constipation, too, but never realised they were all connected. Eventually, when it was all too painful, I told my mum and we went to have my "abscess" removed. When the doctors did this, they realised the lump was soft-tissue cancer and within a week I was a hospital in-patient, miles from home, having intensive chemotherapy. I was fourteen years old.

'At the time of my cancer diagnosis, myself and my family were, understandably, very focused on that, and what I had to do to have the best possible chance of survival. The odds weren't great – only 20 per cent of people in my situation survive more than five years after their diagnosis.

'After eighteen months of chemotherapy and radiotherapy to my pelvis – then six months to see what the long-term effects would be – I was told that my ovaries and uterus had sustained permanent damage, resulting in me now being infertile and essentially in the menopause.

'My oncologist didn't talk to me at length about the menopause or what this would actually mean for me. It was mentioned as a small consequence of my cancer treatment and it didn't sound as if it would have that much impact on me. She prescribed HRT for me, and I went away trusting I had what I needed to get on with my recovery.

'The hard part of getting through my cancer treatment was over. At the time, I was just in survival mode. The idea of my infertility and menopause paled into significance compared with the relief of being alive. The only thing I knew about the menopause was that your periods stopped, which could only be a good thing, right?

'Wrong. But it took me a while to realise this. Over the next two years, I became focused on getting my normal life back, and school exams took over. I was busy and eager to get everything back on track. It eventually took the COVID-19 pandemic and nationwide lockdown to slow me down and make me see what was really going on in my body.

'When my school exams were cancelled, and I stopped to take a breath, only then did I turn my attention to my body and ongoing recovery. I realised I had been struggling and ignoring symptoms for a while – assuming it was just my cancer recovery being a bit slow and problematic. With all the time I had on my hands during lockdown, I thought I may as well learn a bit more about the menopause.

'Lockdown made me join the dots and realise I was menopausal – the tiredness, joint and muscle pains, vaginal atrophy. Up until that point, I had assumed all these problems were hangovers from my cancer treatments years earlier. Even though I was having hot flushes and night sweats, I still hadn't realised I was menopausal.

'Somewhere in my mind, a voice was saying, "But you've survived cancer; you shouldn't complain – you're lucky to be alive." But then I thought, I have to live in this body for the next however many years. I need to take control of it and get the help that I deserve.

'I found Dr Newson and many others on social media. I listened to podcasts and educated myself about the menopause. It made me realise that this is an issue I was allowed to take action on. I thought, Wow, I have actually got an answer as to why my cancer recovery is not going the way I hoped. I don't just have to put up with feeling like this. There is a way to treat it.

'I was previously given a low dose of oestrogen, so that was significantly increased. I also started taking progestogen and testosterone, and was prescribed vaginal oestrogen, too. In only a few months, my symptoms were much better and my future now seems a lot more hopeful than it did before. I feel very lucky to be where I am – to have survived the cancer.

'My perspective on life now helps me have a positive attitude towards my ongoing menopause. I had to learn all about the menopause myself and I now understand how it will affect my body in the future. I had to do this in order to seek out the help I desperately needed.'

Timeout #1: Let's talk about your periods

- Have your periods changed in frequency or stopped altogether?
- Have you noticed any symptoms that could correspond to perimenopause or menopause?
- Are there any reasons your ovarian function might be affected – past treatment, family history, autoimmune condition?
- Have you had an operation to remove your womb and/or your ovaries in the past?
- Have you made an appointment with a healthcare professional to discuss all this?

How are early menopause and POI
investigated and diagnosed?

....

During my undergraduate and postgraduate training, working in hospitals and in general practice, I didn't have any menopause training. I was taught that if a younger woman was worried that her periods had stopped, we should test for pregnancy and, if the test was negative, provide reassurance.

How wrong is that? I can shamefully say it's likely that in my general-practice days I have misdiagnosed many younger women who probably had POI based on that approach. I have seen many young women with irregular periods or periods that stopped and never considered the diagnosis of the menopause or even contemplated the health risks of not treating the menopause in these young women.

Thankfully, awareness is increasing and women are more informed now about the changes in their bodies. More health-care professionals are also being trained and educated about the menopause, including the health risks of not adequately treating the menopause.

If POI or early menopause is suspected, the investigations carried out and the path to diagnosis will likely differ from that of older women, where the diagnosis is based on age and symptoms alone. You will probably need tests and maybe multiple appointments, and I would always recommend trying to see a menopause specialist if you are struggling to get the right diagnosis and treatment.

At your first appointment, your healthcare professional should take a detailed medical history, listen to your story and investigate any symptoms you may be having. If you've had your ovaries removed, then you will not need to have any other tests to make a diagnosis. Many women can be diagnosed on symptoms alone. However, whether you have symptoms or not, you should discuss treatment options, as it is usually important to consider hormones when you are young.

The current NICE and International Menopause Society guidelines are that if you are aged forty to forty-five and early menopause is suspected, blood tests may be useful to confirm a diagnosis. They also state that if you are under forty, hormone blood tests should be done. However, in clinical practice, any hormone blood tests can be unreliable, and I have consulted with many women who have had normal hormone blood tests, but *are* perimenopausal or menopausal. There is no one single reliable test to diagnose POI. Diagnosis is usually made clinically.

So what tests can you expect?

FSH blood test

The test discussed in the menopause guidelines is the FSH test to measure levels of follicle-stimulating hormone (FSH) in the blood. Produced by your brain, FSH stimulates your ovaries to produce oestrogen and testosterone. If your brain notices that your body isn't producing enough oestrogen and/or testosterone, it will start producing more FSH, which is, essentially, its way of saying, 'Come on, we need more hormones.'

FSH levels usually become raised when a woman is menopausal. However, levels can really fluctuate during the menopause, so this test is only a snapshot of the precise moment your blood is taken. While a raised FSH level can sometimes be helpful to know about, a normal or low level doesn't exclude the possibility of you being perimenopausal or menopausal. Some medication (including some psychiatric medication like quetiapine) can actually reduce FSH levels, which then will result in less oestrogen and also testosterone being produced by the ovaries.

Oestradiol

You may have an oestradiol test, which measures the level of oestradiol in the body, but only at the time the blood was taken. Oestradiol levels can vary and change from day to day – even at different times throughout the same day. This means that although oestradiol testing may be used to build up a wider picture, menopause cannot be diagnosed based on this alone.

We often carry out other tests to rule out other conditions. These often include testing to check for diabetes, thyroid-function tests and screening for coeliac disease.

Oestradiol levels can be useful to determine whether you are on the right dose of oestrogen – if you are using oestrogen through the skin as a patch, gel or spray, then levels of oestradiol can usually easily be measured. Younger women often need higher doses of oestrogen compared to older women. It is important to receive enough oestrogen to reduce your symptoms as well as improve your future health.

Tests for testosterone levels are sometimes undertaken before it is prescribed, and they are usually also recommended once you've been prescribed it to ensure that you are having adequate doses.

DEXA scan

Also referred to as a DXA scan, DEXA stands for dual energy X-ray absorptiometry; it is a safe, accurate, painless and non-invasive way of measuring your bone density.

Younger women should have a DEXA scan around the time of diagnosis and, depending on the initial results, it may be repeated. It uses a very low dose of radiation (less than one tenth of the radiation from a chest X-ray, for example), and the scanner calculates the difference between how much radiation enters and exits the bones; the difference represents how much has been absorbed by the bone and other tissues – a measurement known as bone density. As such, it is a measure of quantity rather than quality.

The scanner also uses the bone-density measurement to compare against people of the same age and sex, giving a good indication as to whether you are at risk of, or have already developed, osteoporosis.

A word on the DUTCH test

I've been asked in the past by a number of women about something called the DUTCH test, which stands for dried urine test for comprehensive hormones. This urine test checks for levels of a number of hormones and is sometimes offered by private clinics. However, we don't offer it at my clinic nor recommend it, as I have yet to read enough good-quality evidence about its relevance, and I find the results are often not helpful in making a diagnosis or formulating a treatment plan.

The long-term health risks of an early menopause

Women under the age of forty-five are designed to have hormones. I know that sounds quite radical, but look at it this way: as women, we are designed to have our menopause around the age of fifty or fifty-one. So when the ovaries fail before that age, we are without the oestrogen that others the same age have for longer. We usually need to replace those hormones, and the only way to do that is by taking HRT.

I realise that not everyone wants to take HRT but, if you can, you should absolutely consider taking it when you are young and menopausal (or perimenopausal). The benefits are twofold. Firstly, it will help your symptoms; but secondly – and this is most important if you are younger – it will help your long-term health and reduce your risk of developing various conditions, including heart disease, osteoporosis, type 2 diabetes, clinical depression and dementia. Studies have shown that women who had both their ovaries removed when they were forty years old or younger had an increased risk of developing numerous conditions, including depression, heart disease, type 2 diabetes, arthritis, asthma, dementia and osteoporosis.[121,122,123]

What are the treatment options?
....

As with older women, the most important hormone to replace is oestrogen, and, if you still have a uterus, you will need a progesterone, too. Some women also benefit from taking testosterone.

You can take oestrogen in different ways: via the combined oral contraceptive pill or oestrogen as part of HRT, usually through a patch, gel or spray. The safest type is using 17 beta oestradiol, which is the natural form of oestrogen.

If you have POI, you will tend to need higher doses of oestrogen because this is what we are designed to have when we are younger, so it is important to have enough of it, not only to reduce symptoms, but to protect against disease, too.

If you opt for the combined oral contraceptive pill, remember it is not suitable if you are over thirty-five and smoke, or have a cardiovascular disease or a history of blood clots. In addition, the combined oral contraceptive pills contain synthetic oestrogen and also synthetic progestogens, which actually have more risks (including clot, heart-disease and breast-cancer risks) compared to body-identical HRT. These risks are low in otherwise healthy women.

If you opt for HRT, it can often be a case of trial and error in the first few months to work out how much your body needs – this might be using a couple of patches at once or, like me, a combination of a patch topped up with a gel.

It's important to take oestrogen until at least the usual age of menopause (fifty-one) for the long-term health benefits. Most women continue to take HRT after this age, and it can usually be taken for ever, although the dose may need to change with time.

What are 'normal' ranges of oestrogen?

In most cases, it's beneficial to achieve 'physiological' levels (similar levels to those in women who are still having periods). Generally, this means oestradiol levels above 250 pmol per litre, but some women need more than this to really improve their symptoms. Women do not normally need more than 1,000 pmol per litre.

There is not a maximum 'safe' dose of oestrogen, as women are all different and also they absorb oestrogen in various ways through their skin. This means that two women may be prescribed the same dose but absorb different amounts through their skin into their bloodstream. As oestradiol is an important biologically active hormone in our bodies, it is very safe, so there is no harm in having higher doses. Having too low a dose, however, can lead to you experiencing symptoms and also increase the risk of future disease.

If you still have a uterus, you'll also need a progesterone (either micronised progesterone, a type of progestogen or the Mirena coil). The main advantage of the Mirena coil if you are younger and still having periods is that it also acts as a long-acting contraceptive.

Testosterone

Testosterone production decreases in women with POI and, if your ovaries have been removed or damaged by treatment, you will have even less of it (as your ovaries produce most of it). If you are taking HRT and still feeling like you have low mood, low libido or low energy, speak to a healthcare professional about testosterone.

Lifestyle

As with women going through the menopause in later life, a balanced diet, exercise and mental-health support are also crucial.

What about fertility?

Unless you have had your ovaries removed, it is important to remember there may be a chance of pregnancy when you have POI. This is because ovarian function may return intermittently. We've even had a few surprise pregnancies among our patients!

If you have POI and want to explore fertility options, I

would always recommend speaking to a fertility specialist. Even if you aren't thinking about children right now, it is good to know your options if you change your mind in the future. And it's key to point out that taking HRT is safe if you are trying to conceive.

However, if you want to *avoid* getting pregnant, you need to think about contraception. HRT is not a contraceptive (unless you are using a Mirena coil).

EXPERT VIEW
My experience of POI as both a doctor and a patient – Miss Rebecca Gibbs,
Obstetrics and Gynaecological Consultant and Ambassador for the Daisy Network

Like a lot of younger women I see, Rebecca only discovered she was menopausal while undergoing fertility treatment. Here, she shares the story of her own POI diagnosis, and advice for those who find themselves in a similar situation.

My role working in obstetrics and gynaecology – which covers everything from pregnancy and childbirth to reproductive health – is such a privilege. You see every aspect of being a woman, but it was actually my own experiences that led me towards working more in the area of menopause.

During my training, I didn't learn a lot about menopause; it was something usually handled by colleagues working in general practice and community gynaecology. It was only when I was twenty-nine and my husband and I started trying for a baby that menopause took on a new meaning for me.

I really thought that for a young professional couple we were getting ahead of the game, but it just didn't happen, so we sought medical advice. My periods were pretty normal, but, each time I had blood tests as part of fertility investigations, my FSH levels were higher than before. We decided to have IVF, but every time I was given fertility drugs to stimulate my ovaries into producing eggs, it yielded eggs you would expect of a woman in her forties, not in her twenties.

By my third round of IVF, I was having real menopausal symptoms. I wasn't overly concerned, as some of the hormones you are given during IVF suppress others, so it can give you a taste of what a hot flush feels like. But for me, these symptoms just didn't go away and eventually, I was diagnosed with POI at the age of thirty-one. So here, based on my professional and personal experience, I want to share some practical advice on dealing with a POI diagnosis.

No two POI diagnoses are the same

POI covers an incredibly broad spectrum of experiences, from girls who are diagnosed in their mid-teens, when it is such a huge thing to get your head around, through to women who are thirty-eight or thirty-nine, whose families may be complete and they are at an age when the general conversation around menopause is opening up.

Consider HRT for your future health

Initially, I resisted taking HRT. I had a hard time coming to terms with my diagnosis: one minute I was planning a family, and the next I was being offered HRT, and I found that sudden shift quite brutal.

I'm of the generation who remembers those HRT newspaper headlines [the WHI study linking HRT to breast cancer], and, even as a medical professional who knew the benefits, it took me some time to make up my own mind.

My wake-up call came a few months after my diagnosis when, after deciding to take up roller skating as a hobby, I fell and fractured my wrist. For six weeks, I was unable to deliver babies or scrub in for surgeries; it made me realise how fragile bones could be, and how important oestrogen is in helping to protect against osteoporosis. I now know HRT was the best decision I could have made.

A POI diagnosis can be overwhelming – but remember, HRT will help with any symptoms and replacement should be continued at least until the average age of menopause to protect your heart, bones and brain.

It's so important to have a proper conversation with your chosen healthcare professionals around the benefits and any risks. Ask questions, do your own research. You don't have to rush into a decision; take your time and give it some serious thought.

Find what works for you

If you do decide to take HRT, it's important to find a preparation that works for you. I use oestrogen patches, but if you are a busy twenty-something then the contraceptive pill may be better suited to you – you might already be familiar with it and it might fit in better with your lifestyle; and, of course, it is a form of contraception.

Ask about fertility options

A lot of women, like I did, will come to a POI diagnosis after fertility treatment, so questions about fertility will often be front and centre. But you may not have had a chance to even consider whether children are part of your future plans, or perhaps you had already decided to be child-free.

However you feel right now, it's worth finding out what your options are – such as IVF or egg donation – just in case you change your mind in future.

Don't be afraid to reach out for psychological support

Finding out you have POI can be life-changing. You are contending with the shock of the diagnosis, it may mean the end of an ambition to have a family or you may be concerned about your future health.

I was referred for counselling by my GP after my diagnosis and I found it incredibly helpful.

If you are struggling, I would urge you to speak up. You can ask for a referral from your GP or, if you are already under the care of a specialist clinic, there may be counsellors on the team. Another option is to pay for private counselling.

Unanswered questions? The Daisy Network is here to help

In an ideal world, every woman with POI would have the opportunity to discuss their diagnosis over the course of several appointments, with each appointment looking at a different aspect, from treatment through to fertility and lifestyle advice. But the frustrating reality is that the NHS is so overstretched, and this simply does not always happen. If you have any unanswered questions, that's where the Daisy Network comes in (see Resources, p. 358).

The Daisy Network is a huge source of support for so many women with POI, including live chats with healthcare professionals, resources on getting the most of out of your healthcare appointments and a very supportive community of people who understand what you are going through.

CASE STUDY: POI AND HAVING
A FAMILY – ANNETTE'S STORY

Annette had just turned thirty when she started to experience debilitating fatigue and regular migraines. Soon after, a diagnosis of POI meant that her dream of starting a family seemed out of reach – until she made the decision to adopt as a single parent.

'A decade ago, I'd just hit my thirties and life was pretty good – but there was one problem. I was unbearably tired and falling asleep on the sofa at 6pm every evening because it was impossible to fight the overwhelming fatigue. I also started getting migraines like clockwork every month.

'At first, I put this down to my stressful job. I was working in international events and having a busy time working on lots of different projects and travelling across time zones. As I was single, with very little time for a relationship, I decided to take a break from the contraceptive pill to see if that would stop the migraines. But three months later, I felt even worse – I was absolutely exhausted, had started having hot flushes and hadn't had a period since I stopped taking the pill. In hindsight, it's clear that the pill had been compensating for my lack of hormones.

'I made an appointment to see my family doctor, who was sure that it was nothing to worry about. But he explained that in rare cases it could mean an early menopause, so he ordered some tests just to be sure. He assured me that this was very unusual, so I wasn't especially worried.

'I was shocked, then, when my results came in: my thyroid levels were in serious decline and my levels of oestrogen and FSH weren't what they should have been. I was prescribed thyroxine immediately (which I'll need to take for the rest of my life) and

199

referred to an endocrinologist and gynaecologist for further investigations.

'I'd always assumed that having my first ultrasound scan would be a magical moment where I'd get to see my baby for the first time, while a supportive partner held my hand. Instead, I found myself scared and alone in a hospital waiting room, waiting to find out what was wrong, surrounded by expectant mothers.

'Then, after lots of poking and prodding, I was diagnosed with POI – basically, an early menopause. I sat in the gynaecologist's office in absolute disbelief, feeling my heart break with every word she spoke. It hit me that the future I had planned was crumbling into oblivion, and she handed me a box of tissues as the tears started to flow.

'POI and infertility are often considered to be part and parcel of the same condition, but that's not necessarily the case. Some people with POI may still have irregular or infrequent periods and may even be able to conceive. But, in some cases – like mine – POI can lead to periods stopping altogether, resulting in infertility.

'After my diagnosis, I just wanted to hide away. Dealing with the emotional fallout was so much harder than fixing the physical symptoms. But, after about six months, I decided that it was time to investigate my options. A doctor explained that the only way for me to carry a baby to full term would be through egg donation. This would need to be privately funded, as the NHS in the UK doesn't offer this treatment to single people.

'I investigated IVF privately but, with costs of around £10,000, it was out of my reach. So, I decided to concentrate on work and put aside any thoughts of having a family of my own. As a result, I started to push people away. I had started dating again, but I struggled with how to explain my diagnosis to a potential partner. And whenever I was invited to a baby shower, christening or a child's birthday party, I'd come away feeling sad and deflated.

'Finally, two years after my diagnosis, I accepted that I really wanted to be a mum. That's when I decided to look at other options. For me, adoption was the obvious choice, and I made the terrifying decision to adopt as a single parent. Going through the adoption process alone was isolating at times, but I had an amazing support network, and I met some incredible people who were going through the same process.

'After going in front of a panel, I was finally approved as an adopter, but it took five more months and two failed matches before I was united with a six-month-old baby – my son. He came home with me a month later, and six months after that we officially became a family in the eyes of the courts.

'It's now almost ten years since my diagnosis of POI, and I'm mum to a bright and active son, who I believe I was destined to have in my life. My journey to motherhood wasn't easy or conventional, but it gave me the strength I needed to become the woman I am today. Some people talk about menopause being the end of a chapter – but for me it was just the beginning.'

8

Menopause and Cancer

Four things you will learn in this chapter:

1. How cancer treatments can result in an earlier menopause

2. The typical symptoms you may experience

3. Treatment options: weighing up the benefits and risks

4. Spotlight on breast cancer

At the time of a cancer diagnosis, there is a lot of information to process. The primary focus will – and should – be successfully treating your cancer. Other considerations are unlikely to be a priority at this point – but what about life beyond cancer?

Globally, the number of people diagnosed with cancer per year will exceed 23 million by 2030.[124] Breast cancer is the most common cancer in women, accounting for more than 25 per cent of new cancer cases each year. Earlier diagnosis and advances in treatment mean that breast cancer now has an excellent prognosis, and 90 per cent of women become long-term survivors. This increases to 99 per cent of women, if diagnosed with early, localised breast cancer.[125]

Once treatment has been completed, people who have had the disease then start on another journey, which is that of living with a personal history of cancer. Although many of them will thankfully be 'cancer free', this does not mean, necessarily, that they are free of symptoms related to their illness or their treatment for it.[126] Being a menopausal woman who has had breast cancer and not receiving individualised advice and treatment can be very isolating and frightening.

Despite my platform, I'm a pretty shy person. Writing about my family and my own menopause journey in this book wasn't a decision I took lightly, believe me. It's been a challenging, yet hugely cathartic process, and I hope reading about my experiences has been helpful to you as a reader.

What's more, having firmly moved out of my comfort zone to write about my personal life, I then found writing this chapter the most challenging part of the entire process.

Why? Because I absolutely wanted to get it right.

I know women with a history of cancer, or those undergoing active treatment right now, are often frustrated at the wider menopause conversation. Or, to be more specific, the fact that they are so often excluded from the conversation in the media, in social media and in the consulting room alike. And it is these frustrations that lead women to contact me, whether as patients at my clinic, hanging back to talk to me after a speaking engagement or in a midnight message via social media.

So I wanted this chapter to be a chance to include you all in the menopause conversation, with clear information and advice that you can take back and discuss with your healthcare team. It will give you a roadmap, explaining why your menopause may be earlier than you expected, the types of symptoms you may experience and the available treatments (both hormonal and non-hormonal).

How does cancer affect my menopause?

Many women experience an early menopause as a consequence of the treatment they receive for cancer, which can include chemotherapy, radiotherapy to the pelvic area or removal of the ovaries. Some medication – for example, tamoxifen and aromatase inhibitors (see p. 222) – can also cause an early menopause. In addition, medications that turn off ovarian function, such as Goserelin, usually also lead to menopause occurring.

Just like with a natural menopause, your menopause will be unique to you. No one can predict what symptoms you'll have or how you will feel. You may sail through it and have no symptoms or barely noticeable ones; or you may feel like a completely different person and battle on a daily basis with a range of symptoms that are physical, emotional and psychological.

In my clinical experience, many women fall somewhere in between. Whether you experience symptoms or not, there are still health risks (such as increased future risk of heart disease, osteoporosis, type 2 diabetes and dementia) as a result of low hormone levels.[127]

It is not unusual for women to be told by their cancer-care team that menopause may be a consequence of their treatment, but, because the focus at that point is on cancer treatment and survival, very little further discussion is had. It is often only when treatment has finished, and women try to return to their 'normal' lives, that they start to understand what the menopause is going to mean for them.

However, many women do not recall any mention at all of menopause as a possible issue that may arise from their breast-cancer treatment. This can mean that they attribute the symptoms they experience to their treatment instead. For example, many have told me they thought their anxiety, depression, joint pains and brain fog were a result of having breast cancer or due to their chemotherapy, rather than their menopause.

You might find that treatment may stop your periods for a while and then they return, or it can be a permanent loss of periods and you will remain post-menopausal for the rest of your life.

If you're recovering from surgery or undergoing cancer treatment, it can be difficult to tell which symptoms are side effects of this and which are due to the menopause, caused by a lack of hormones. Fatigue and joint pain, for example, are common to both. This is why the menopause can sometimes creep up on you without you being fully aware of what's really going on in your body.

Given the increasing numbers of women with a history of breast cancer who are both struggling to cope with their menopausal symptoms and carrying an increased risk to their future cardiovascular and bone health, it is imperative that they are able to access appropriate support and are given the most up-to-date and evidence-based information regarding their options. And this should be via a healthcare professional with a specialist interest in the menopause.

The following are some of the signs and symptoms of both cancer treatment and the menopause that may overlap:

No periods

Cancer treatments like chemotherapy can cause irregular periods, so you may notice a change to the frequency or flow. Once everything has settled down after treatment, if you are still bleeding or start bleeding in an unusual, heavy or prolonged way, especially if you are taking tamoxifen, talk to your doctor or a healthcare professional about it. Many women find their periods stop, and, even if this is a direct result of cancer treatments, it is indicative of low hormone levels.

Hot flushes and night sweats

These can also be a side effect of hormonal therapies, often used to treat breast cancer and sometimes womb or ovarian cancer. However, if they persist, they are more likely to be related to the menopause.

Night sweats

Sweating can be a symptom of cancer or may be due to cancer treatment. But again, if the sweats persist, you should consider whether they are related to your hormones.

Mood changes and anxiety

Hormone deficiency can cause symptoms such as irritability, low or anxious mood, tearfulness and low self-esteem – a whole range of emotions. It's often the symptom that bothers people the most, as it can make you feel so unlike your usual self. These feelings can also be a normal reaction to your diagnosis and treatments for cancer, and in the adjustment phase afterwards.

Cancer will undoubtedly cause you to feel anxious at times and worried about possible effects of treatments, the impact on your partner or family and friends and the future – and these are all entirely understandable. The menopause can also increase feelings of anxiety considerably, exacerbating the worries you already have. This might include concerns about treatment for your menopausal symptoms, such as taking HRT.

Fatigue and poor sleep

Fatigue and exhaustion are common when recovering from cancer and may also be symptoms of menopause. It's also not unusual for sleep to be affected by menopause, either due to night sweats, needing to go to the toilet, feeling anxious or stressed or a whole host of other possible reasons.

Brain fog

You may be familiar with 'chemo brain'; well, brain fog is the menopause equivalent. A lack of hormones can cause memory lapses, poor concentration, difficulty absorbing information and a feeling that your brain is like cotton wool. Brain fog can be a real challenge, particularly at work, and it can affect the simplest of tasks, like reading a book, listening to a podcast or following the plot in a film.

Joint pains

Joint pains can often be a side effect of a group of medications called aromatase inhibitors, which are a common treatment for breast cancer. However, as oestrogen and testosterone work as anti-inflammatories in your muscles and joints, when levels fall during the menopause, many women find that pains in those areas are common menopausal symptoms, too.

Hair and skin changes

Cancer treatments can lead to dry, itchy or even scaly skin, hair thinning and hair loss. However, as mentioned on p. 166 and 176, these are also common menopausal symptoms.

Vaginal and urinary symptoms

Genitourinary symptoms are very common during the meno-pause and can lead to pain, discomfort and irritation. Some treatments for cancer can lead to worsening of these things. For example, radiotherapy to the vagina (or surrounding tissues) can exacerbate vaginal dryness, while radiotherapy to the pelvic area can irritate the bladder or urinary tract.

Sexual-function problems

Hormone fluctuations during the perimenopause and meno-pause can lead to low libido. And even if you do feel in the mood, physical symptoms such as vaginal dryness can make having sex painful.

Cancer treatments can also have a negative impact on sex and rela-tionships for a multitude of reasons. These include poor self-esteem and perception of body image, fatigue, stress and anxiety, and symptoms of hormone deficiency, such as low libido and vaginal dryness that can, again, make having sex painful and uncomfortable.

For women who have had cancer in the past, treatment-related sexual dysfunction is, unfortunately, one of the most prevalent and distressing side effects and is often not addressed and managed adequately.[128] All types of cancer treatment (surgery, radiotherapy, chemotherapy and hormonal therapy) have the potential to negatively impact sexual function. For women who have had surgery, the consequences may be obvious, or much less apparent, such as nerve damage or permanent loss of sensation.[129]

Timeout #1: Recently diagnosed with cancer? Questions you may want to ask

Take a few minutes to think about the questions you may want to ask at your next appointment:

- Will my treatment mean that I will go through an early menopause?
- How soon after treatment starts should I expect menopausal symptoms (if any)?
- What treatments are available?
- Is there any information I can take away with me today to read over?

Advice on dealing with menopause following a cancer diagnosis

Knowing about possible menopause symptoms helps you to understand more about the effects of hormone deficiency and to figure out what is a consequence of your cancer treatment and what might be caused by the menopause. For many women, their quality of life is really negatively affected by their menopause, and this should not be underestimated.

As well as the changes just described, there are some long-term effects of the menopause that it's important to be aware of. After the menopause, women live with hormone deficiency for the rest of their lives. When it comes to a lack of oestrogen, the two biggest potential impacts on your health in the future are osteoporosis and cardiovascular disease (see pp. 97–101), while research has shown that the menopause can also increase the risk of other conditions, including type 2 diabetes, dementia and clinical depression.[130] Other long-term impacts can include vaginal dryness and issues with sex and intimacy as well as fertility.

What positive steps can I take?

It's important to take a holistic view to managing your menopause, particularly if you are undergoing or have recently finished cancer treatment. Taking this broad approach is usually best, as there is no single 'right' way to tackle the menopause; just bear in mind that it can affect your physical and mental health and how you feel will vary from day to day. Your decisions regarding treatments may evolve with time, too – what you decide now may be very different to what you want to do in several years' time. It is perfectly fine to change your mind regarding treatment choices.

- **Rest up.** As many as nine out of ten people undergoing cancer treatment experience fatigue, and, as we know, this can be a menopause symptom, too.[131] Try to keep a consistent sleeping routine where possible.[132]

- **Prioritise your mental health.** Research shows that anxiety and depression affect people with cancer (up to 10 and 20 per cent respectively), and they are also common in the menopause.[133] Speak to your healthcare team about accessing mental-health support; a number of cancer charities (for example, the gynaecological charity the Eve Appeal and Macmillan Cancer Support) run advice services. At home, try writing a diary to help you feel more in control of your emotions and thoughts, practise breathing and relaxation techniques daily and find supportive friends and be open with them about how you're feeling. Make time for getting outdoors.

- **Stay active.** Exercise is not only important for your general health, but also helps to keep your bones and heart strong and can be a significant part of cancer recovery. Exercise can also reduce breast cancer risk.[134] Always consult your healthcare team before embarking on a new exercise regime, but, if cleared to do so, aim for a mixture of activities that raise your heart rate and also impact your joints – like running or high-intensity interval-training (HIIT) workouts. If cancer-related fatigue or joint pains are a factor, start with a lower-impact activity that is slow and gentle, and gradually build up the duration and frequency. It will do wonders for your emotional wellbeing and mental health, too.

- **Eat well.** You may have already made efforts to eat a healthy diet when you were going through your cancer treatment and recovery. Foods that are important for menopause are those that are rich in calcium and vitamin D (for your bones), pre- and probiotics (friendly to the gut), carbohydrates with a low glycaemic index (GI) that are broken down more slowly and keep you fuller for longer and foods rich in omega-3 oils for brain health.

- **Make adjustments at work.** Whether you go out to work or work from home, it's helpful to tell someone if there are any symptoms relating to menopause and/or cancer treatment that you are finding tricky to manage. You may need to adapt your workspace, get a fan or sit near a window, take more frequent mental pitstops or break up tasks differently. These little things can make a big difference to your comfort, focus and productivity levels.

What are my treatment options?

At the heart of good menopause care is the belief that it should be individualised. When you've had a cancer diagnosis, conversations around menopause treatment can feel confusing and, at times, overwhelming. Do you take HRT or not? Will medications interfere with each other? And who is the best person to talk to – your family doctor, your cancer team or a menopause specialist? My advice here would be to start with the health professional you feel most comfortable with and take it from there.

I'm now going to take you through various treatment options. This is designed to be used as a guide, but the key thing here is to keep talking to your own healthcare professionals, because they will know your circumstances and can help; some people need to see several before they find one who fully understands how they are feeling and who will also discuss the harm in *not* giving treatment, as well as any benefits and risks of having it.

Vaginal hormonal treatments

As oestrogen is important in your vulva, vagina and surrounding urinary tract, the majority of menopausal women who have had cancer experience localised symptoms. These include vaginal dryness, soreness, irritation, urinary frequency, urinary incontinence and urinary-tract infections.

There are non-hormonal vaginal moisturisers and lubricants, which can be beneficial for some women.[135] However, the optimal treatment is restoring the low hormones in these tissues.[136] Women can usually use vaginal hormonal preparations following any cancer diagnosis, and they will really improve menopausal genitourinary symptoms. The hormone dose is very low, and absorption into your bloodstream is minimal, so vaginal hormone preparations can be used even by women who have been advised not to take systemic HRT.[137]

Non-hormonal treatments

It's important to explore all possibilities with your healthcare team and find treatment options to suit your circumstances and wishes. Whether you decide to take HRT or not, be sure to consider your menopause holistically, as mentioned, looking at ways to boost your nutrition, exercise and general wellbeing, too.

Lifestyle

Reducing or stopping alcohol, increasing exercise and optimising nutrition can be really beneficial to your future health – both physical and mental. Some women find that lifestyle changes can also improve and lessen menopausal symptoms.[138] I will be covering exercise and nutrition in more detail in Chapters 10 and 11.

Cognitive behavioural therapy (CBT)

CBT is a talking therapy that can help you to manage your problems by changing the way you think and behave. There is some evidence that it can improve some menopausal symptoms, including vasomotor ones (hot flushes and night sweats), low mood and anxiety, as well as sleep disturbances.[139,140]

Prescribed medications

There are medications that can be prescribed to women, but side effects can often limit their usefulness. Studies have shown that they can improve hot flushes and night sweats, and they can sometimes improve mood changes, too.[141] They include the following:

- **Antidepressants.** Selective serotonin reuptake inhibitors (SSRIs) are the most commonly prescribed antidepressants. They can improve symptoms of moderate to severe depression by increasing levels of serotonin in your brain. There is also some evidence that they improve hot flushes and night sweats due to the menopause. Escitalopram and venlafaxine seem to be the most effective antidepressants when used in this way.[142] However, there needs to be some caution for women taking tamoxifen. Tamoxifen is a 'prodrug', which means that after it is taken, it needs to be 'activated' or converted into its active form (endoxifen) by a liver enzyme called CYP2D6. Some antidepressants inhibit the function of this enzyme – so those which are strong inhibitors (fluoxetine, bupropion and paroxetine) should be avoided in women who are also taking tamoxifen; alternatives such as sertraline, citalopram, escitalopram and venlafaxine are usually preferable.[143] Many women who take antidepressants when they do not have clinical depression find that side effects such as sleep disturbance, sexual dysfunction and weight gain limit their use.[144]

- **Gabapentin.** Usually prescribed for conditions such as epilepsy and migraine, studies show that gabapentin can help with hot flushes.[145,146] Side effects can include drowsiness, dry mouth and weight gain.
- **Pregabalin.** A drug to treat anxiety and epilepsy, pregabalin has a similar effect to gabapentin; it can be better tolerated, but many women still experience side effects.

I've had cancer. Can I take HRT?

Many healthcare professionals and women are worried about the perceived risks of causing a cancer recurrence or progression if they prescribe or are given HRT (please note, breast cancer and HRT are discussed later in this chapter – see pp. 222–31).

Clearly, advising women not to take HRT should be a decision that is made after reviewing the cancer-specific risks associated with taking it, versus the benefits in terms of quality of life and prevention of long-term conditions such as cardiovascular disease, osteoporosis, type 2 diabetes and dementia. Young women who are menopausal at an early age have an increased risk of other conditions, too, such as lung and kidney disease and mental-health problems, which can be reduced by taking HRT.[147]

In addition, it is well known that refusal of HRT decreases not only quality of life, but also the life expectancy of young menopausal patients by several years. In one study, this was found to be two years lost over a seventeen-year follow-up period, mainly due to increased death from cardiovascular disease and also osteoporosis.[148] It's crucial that any decision not to prescribe HRT is not made without justification and full discussion with the patient involved, as this could potentially lead to harm.

The evidence regarding HRT following many types of cancer is weak or the studies have not been done, and the decision whether to take it or not should be tailored to the individual, after discussion with the cancer specialist, if appropriate.

Many traditional contraindications to hormone replacement therapy (HRT) are based on the theoretical potential for HRT to worsen a disease process and rarely on supporting data. The presence of oestrogen receptors in a cancer does not mean that these cancers have been caused by oestrogen; nor does it mean that oestrogen is contraindicated as a treatment. As mentioned before, women have cells all over their bodies with oestrogen receptors on them.

For example, there are many types of cancer that are not related to female hormones, and women who have had them in the past are likely to benefit, without increasing their risks, from taking HRT. These include most types of lymphomas, leukaemias, thyroid, kidney, bowel, liver, bladder, lung and stomach cancers.

HRT can be considered for any woman who has debilitating menopausal symptoms that impact negatively on her quality of life. Tailoring of the product, dose, route and regimen may avoid some of the theoretical risks of HRT in particular women.

HRT is effective at relieving a whole host of symptoms, which will usually improve within three to six months of starting treatment. These include the physical ones, like hot flushes, joint aches and fatigue, and psychological ones, like low mood, anxiety, loss of confidence and mood swings. The risk of developing osteoporosis reduces, as the bones will be protected from weakening through lack of oestrogen. In addition, the risk of cardiovascular disease reduces, making the development of heart problems, stroke or vascular dementia less likely. Those who take HRT also have a lower future risk of type 2 diabetes, osteoarthritis, bowel cancer and clinical depression.[149]

Spotlight on gynaecological cancers and HRT

Each year in the UK, more than 22,000 women are diagnosed with a gynaecological cancer – womb, ovarian, cervical, vulval and vaginal.[150] If you have had a diagnosis of a gynaecological cancer, you may be wondering what your treatment options are. Let's look at this in some more detail:

Ovarian cancer

As with many of the cancers, there are not enough data to fully reassure women that there is no increased risk of ovarian cancer recurrence with the use of HRT after diagnosis and treatment, but, having said that, there are no convincing data to deny HRT either.[151]

Several studies have shown that taking HRT after ovarian cancer does not increase recurrence of the cancer (in some studies, it even significantly increases the overall survival of patients).[152,153,154]

Many women who have had ovarian cancer will have had a hysterectomy at the same time as a bilateral oophorectomy (an operation to remove both ovaries). This then makes hormone-replacement options easier, as progesterone is not usually then needed.

Womb cancer

Treatment for this type of cancer is usually surgery, via a hysterectomy and oophorectomy. Unlike some other types of cancer, womb cancer is usually diagnosed early, meaning it is generally confined to the womb and surgery tends to be curative.

The concern about HRT after womb cancer is that oestrogen-only HRT reactivates any unsuspected endometrial cancer cells that escaped before surgery. Because of this, many specialists prefer to prescribe combined continuous HRT for women with a history of womb cancer.[155]

Reassuringly, there are some studies that show no decrease in survival with use of HRT in women after womb cancer, and/or data that contraindicate the use of HRT after womb cancer.[156,157]

Other gynaecological cancers

Most other gynaecological cancers are not related to hormones.[158] This means that HRT for women after cervical, vulval or vaginal cancers should not be contraindicated.[159]

Additionally, women can still usually use vaginal hormonal preparations following any cancer diagnosis, which will really improve menopausal genitourinary symptoms (see p. 213 for more information).[160]

As with many other areas of menopause research, there are no long-term, randomised trials of HRT after different types of cancers.

A fully informed patient should be empowered and supported to make a decision that best balances benefits to that individual when weighed against potential risks. It is their right to be involved in making choices about their future care and treatment.

As menopause specialists, we usually talk with our patients about what is known and unknown and give each individual patient the option of HRT, based on their own individual benefits and any potential risks, even though the pharmaceutical industry and licensing agencies have opted out of the clinical dilemma or even deemed their type of cancer a 'contraindication' for taking HRT.

In addition, NICE guidance states that the impact of severe menopausal symptoms on quality of life may be substantial, and some women for whom HRT is contraindicated may choose to accept a degree of risk that might be considered by some to outweigh its benefits.[161]

Other treatments

Around half of perimenopausal and menopausal women worldwide seek assistance from complementary and alternative medicine approaches, including herbal medicines, massage therapy and acupuncture for symptomatic relief.[162]

There is some evidence that acupuncture can be beneficial for some women.[163] And there are also lots of herbal preparations marketed to help menopausal symptoms, such as hot flushes. While there is no good-quality evidence to support the use of herbal medicines, the lack of evidence does not mean that they can't be beneficial in some women.

NICE guidance on menopause diagnosis and management says women with a history of (or at high risk of) breast cancer should be advised that although there is some evidence that St John's wort may be of benefit in the relief of symptoms like hot flushes, there is uncertainty about appropriate doses, persistence of effect, variation in the nature and potency of preparations and potential serious interactions with other drugs. (Note: St John's wort should be avoided if you are taking tamoxifen.[164])

If you do decide to try herbal medicines, always speak to a healthcare professional beforehand. Make sure you know all the ingredients of any product that you take; and, if you aren't feeling any better after taking it for three months, it is unlikely to work.

CASE STUDY: MENOPAUSE AFTER A CERVICAL
CANCER DIAGNOSIS – EMMA'S STORY

Emma was just thirty and a new mother when she was diagnosed with cervical cancer. Like a lot of women with a new diagnosis of cancer, menopause wasn't a focus in those early weeks of her treatment, so she felt unprepared for the symptoms she had.

'In 2014, five months after the birth of my daughter, I was diagnosed with cervical cancer.

'I was told that my treatment would force me into an early menopause, and that it would probably take about a year to happen. I don't think I appreciated what that actually meant. We didn't learn anything about menopause at school, so I wasn't prepared for the symptoms when they came.

'As it happened, it only took two months for me to go into full-blown menopause. I can still remember my first hot flush; I was at the hospital having treatment when this huge wave of heat came out of nowhere. The hot flushes were the worst part for me; I honestly thought I was going to combust at times.

'I started HRT, but I felt awful. For months, I had severe migraines every single day, which were debilitating; at one point, I was convinced I had a brain tumour. It's no exaggeration to say that I found the menopause symptoms harder to cope with than my cancer treatment.

'I started doing my own research and got a second opinion about my HRT. I changed how I take it, and this has changed my life. I never suffer with hot flushes or migraines, and I feel super. It has taken me a long time to get to this point and understand my body and hormone levels.

'I have never been embarrassed about entering menopause so early, I embrace it and see the positives in it.'

Spotlight on breast cancer

Let's start with a quick look at breast cancer and how it links to hormones.

Breast cancer is the second-most common type of cancer in the UK and around one in seven women will develop it over their lifetime.

Thankfully, in the UK, breast-cancer survival has doubled in the last forty years. It is a complex disease, and there are many different types. The role of oestrogen is still poorly understood. When cancerous cells are examined after a biopsy or surgery, it's established whether or not they have receptors for oestrogen. If they do, it's known as oestrogen-receptor-positive (ER-positive) breast cancer; if they don't, it's ER-negative. This is important when it comes to deciding on treatments for menopause symptoms. So knowing whether your cancer was ER positive or negative may influence your decision about taking HRT – or not.

Aromatase inhibitors and tamoxifen

Tamoxifen is a type of hormone therapy used for the prevention and treatment of breast cancer. It is a selective oestrogen receptor modulator (SERM), which means it blocks oestrogen on some cells, including in the breast, but not on others. Tamoxifen is used in both pre- and post-menopausal women to treat breast cancer. Interestingly, studies have shown that pre-menopausal women who take tamoxifen actually have a higher level (around three to ten times higher) of oestradiol in their bodies compared to women who do not.[165] These studies highlight that treatment with tamoxifen is not as simple as 'switching off' oestrogen in the body, and allowing post-menopausal women to have some oestrogen in the form of HRT to treat menopausal symptoms is unlikely to be harmful. Many specialists feel more reassured giving HRT to women who are also taking tamoxifen.

Aromatase inhibitors are used to treat breast cancer in post-menopausal women whose ovaries are no longer producing oestrogen. Sometimes they are used in those who are pre-menopausal, but usually only if their ovaries are 'switched off', which is usually done with a hormone injection. The purpose of taking aromatase inhibitors is to prevent the production of oestrogen anywhere in the body.

If you are taking an aromatase inhibitor and experiencing dreadful symptoms, you could talk to your breast specialist about the possibility of either stopping your medication for a few weeks to see if this improves your menopausal symptoms or taking tamoxifen or an alternative instead.

Hormonal treatments and breast cancer

You may have made all the right changes to your lifestyle and tried non-hormonal treatments. However, these may not be enough to improve all your menopause symptoms. Or you may want to consider taking HRT for future health benefits.

It's common for women with a personal history of breast cancer who come to my clinic to be concerned about their future risk of osteoporosis or dementia as a consequence of their low hormones. Women also self-refer because they simply don't feel listened to or empowered to have a say in their menopause care.

Women will say they have simply been told they are not 'allowed' to take HRT – that taking it would never be an option for them – and that is the end of the conversation.

As one woman who responded to our survey put it: 'I have had my breast cancer treatment – right mastectomy, reconstruction, lymph-node removal, left-side lumpectomy and chemo; and now someone was dictating how I had to live the rest of my life.'

It is essential that women are central to any decision-making process regarding taking HRT – or any other treatment, for that matter (and I'll be outlining some tips on getting the best out of menopause conversations with your doctor and other healthcare professionals at the end of this chapter).

NICE guidance on early and locally advanced breast cancer states HRT should not be routinely recommended to women with menopausal symptoms and a history of breast cancer.[166]

In exceptional circumstances, it adds that HRT can be offered to women with severe menopausal symptoms and with whom the associated risks have been discussed. This guidance must take into account the type of breast cancer and the patient's symptoms; if I have a patient in front of me saying that their quality of life is terrible, I owe it to them to have a detailed conversation.

Studies designed to evaluate the safety of HRT in breast-cancer survivors have yielded conflicting results, and there is a lack of good-quality, robust evidence to guide us. Most of the studies are small and of short duration and have only looked at the effect of synthetic hormones, rather than the body-identical hormones that are usually prescribed today. Overall, the evidence is reassuring, and most of the studies have not demonstrated an increased risk of breast-cancer recurrence or death.[167] The HABITS (Hormonal Replacement Therapy After Breast Cancer – Is It Safe?) study is the only study to have demonstrated a very small increased risk of recurrence in some women, but there was no increased risk of dying from breast cancer in women who took HRT after having it.[168] In addition, the set-up of this study has been criticised – women who entered it did not have a baseline mammogram.

What is key is that all treatment decisions are based on your individual circumstances, and, if you decide that you may want to take hormonal treatment, this should be a shared decision-making process between you, your cancer team and a menopause specialist.

EXPERT VIEW
Key barriers to good menopause care for women with a history of breast cancer – Dr Alison Macbeth

Dr Alison is a GP with a special interest in women's health, and for the past eight years has worked as a speciality doctor in an NHS breast clinic. She diagnoses and treats women with breast cancer, as well as providing care to those with a high-risk family history of breast cancer. She is also an accredited menopause specialist who runs a menopause clinic within NHS breast services, providing evidence-based holistic care.

For me, one of the main barriers to good menopause care for women with a history of breast cancer is lack of access to menopause specialists with specific breast-disease training.

Helping women with a history of breast cancer through the menopause is complex, and I can see the issues from a range of angles – as a GP, as a breast doctor and as a menopause specialist.

Understandably for such a specialised area, GPs will often struggle, and often seek advice from the patient's breast-cancer specialist. Yet neither breast surgeons nor breast oncologists have specific training in menopause, so GPs are often left without the guidance they are looking for.

And what about the patients themselves? When it comes to menopause, more often than not, women turn to Dr Google for help. This is in marked contrast to when they undergo their initial cancer treatments. Then, patients are looked after by whole teams of surgeons, nurses and oncologists; but when that acute treatment is over, things look very different. They switch from a face-to-face annual review by the breast surgeons' team to a virtual follow-up, where they are simply sent for an annual mammogram, followed up by a letter giving them their results.

This can lead to a sense of abandonment and offers little opportunity to talk about any problems they may not have thought related to their cancer treatment, such as vaginal dryness or mood disorders.

I see patients every day who have 'survived' their initial treatment and thought the hardest part was over, and don't understand why they are struggling now. They are often made to feel guilty for complaining about their menopause symptoms, and that they should just be happy to be alive. I see women who feel they should just accept they haven't been able to have sex with their partners for years since treatment, they have lost their jobs and their marriages have collapsed due to their symptoms.

If I could give one piece of advice to any woman reading this who is in a similar situation, I would urge you not to stay quiet and accept this as your lot – because it isn't.

Keep a diary of your symptoms; contact your breast-care nurse. There is much we can do for most of your symptoms and your life is not over. Treatment strategies are very individual, so what works for one woman may be different for another.

More training is required for breast teams in menopause care, and it's vitally important that women can access advice in a timely manner, rather than be held for up to two years on a waiting list to see a menopause specialist. I believe every breast unit should have access to a breast-trained menopause specialist (but then I am biased).

Don't suffer in silence. There are many tweaks and changes we can offer to make you feel like 'you' again.

SURVEY: EXPERIENCES OF WOMEN SEEKING MENOPAUSE CARE AFTER BREAST CANCER

Menopause care for women with a personal history of breast cancer remains a really neglected area, due to the controversy around the role of hormones in the disease. But what are the experiences of women who do seek help for menopause after a breast-cancer diagnosis?

In 2022, Dr Sarah Ball along with Newson Health launched an online survey for clinic patients with a history of breast cancer to find out their experiences, particularly when it came to accessing advice and treatment. We received responses from 168 women. So, what did we find?

Three quarters of respondents said that after their cancer diagnosis, menopause was not even mentioned as a possible consequence of their treatment. 'I was unaware that all the other symptoms I had were due to the menopause: I thought the anxiety, depression and myriad other symptoms were down to having had breast cancer,' one respondent said. 'Chemotherapy threw me into the menopause severely, which I was not warned about,' said another.

The effect of menopause symptoms on these women was profound: a third (36 per cent) said they had a severe impact on their career, 40 per cent reported a severe impact on their relationships and 62 per cent said menopause had affected their overall quality of life.

When it came to discussing the issue of menopause with healthcare professionals, the picture was mixed. Almost three quarters (73 per cent) said they felt unable to raise the issue of menopause care with their breast surgical team, compared to 70 per cent with their cancer team and 52 per cent with their GP.

Only 19 per cent of respondents had been referred to an NHS menopause clinic, and the vast majority (94 per cent) had not received any written information about the menopause.

Four out of five (80 per cent) felt relatively or completely uninvolved in decisions about their menopause. 'My consultant advised me that he felt very uncomfortable prescribing HRT but said that if life became unbearable and I was about to shoot my husband, then we could have a conversation about it,' one respondent said.

Though a small survey, this is an important one. It underscores the impact menopause symptoms can have on quality of life for women living with cancer, and lays bare the sheer lack of menopause information shared with women following their cancer diagnosis. At the very time they need guidance – when what they desperately need is up-front information, a personalised conversation and the right to a say in their care – many are being made to feel confused and isolated.

Helping your genital and urinary symptoms

Your vagina, vulva and surrounding tissues need oestrogen to function well. Many breast-cancer treatments suppress women's own oestrogen, which can result in troublesome symptoms. These (in addition to the menopause) can be so severe in some women that normal daily activities are affected, including sitting, walking and wearing certain clothing and underwear, as well as sleep.

While many menopausal symptoms often improve over the years, those of GSM (genitourinary syndrome of menopause) tend to worsen with time. Try to avoid using soap, shower gels, deodorants or 'intimate' products on the area; instead, use a gentle emollient wash, such as Cetraben®. Panty liners, spermicides and many brands of lubricants can contain irritants and should be avoided. Tight-fitting clothing and long-term use of sanitary pads or synthetic materials can also worsen symptoms.

Vaginal moisturisers such as YES®VM, Sylk Intimate, or Regelle® can help to hydrate your tissues and reduce soreness and discomfort throughout the day. Specialist lubricants for when having sex, such as Sylk, YES®OB or YES®WB, can ease discomfort and make the experience more enjoyable. If you are using a barrier method of contraception, water-based lubricants are usually best.

Non-hormonal treatments may not be enough to manage severe symptoms, however, and this is where you should discuss the option of using local vaginal oestrogen or other vaginal hormonal treatments. Most women who have had breast cancer in the past can still use vaginal hormonal preparations, as they are not absorbed into your body and the doses are very low.[169]

If you do decide to try vaginal oestrogen, don't be put off by the information that is packaged with your medication; it is not correct and should be rectified. In fact, the All-Party Parliamentary Group on Menopause (a group of MPs who were tasked with looking into the menopause) have called on the government to work with the MHRA to update information for patients and healthcare professionals but, frustratingly, at the time of writing this hasn't happened.[170]

CASE STUDY: VAGINAL OESTROGEN AFTER A BREAST-CANCER DIAGNOSIS – MEL'S STORY

Mel decided to try vaginal oestrogen several years after her breast-cancer treatment finished.

'I recently made the decision to start using vaginal oestrogen. Enough was enough.

'My symptoms were so severe and worsening, and it was really impacting my quality of life. For me, it has been a great decision and has made a huge difference.

'However, I don't regret not making the decision earlier, as I believe you have to make each decision in life based on the information available and how you feel at the time – you can't look back with regret.

'My point is, things can change, the balance can be tipped and that's ok. The most important thing is being comfortable that it is the right decision for you. I can truly understand why women who have had breast cancer may choose to either have or not have HRT, either vaginally or systemically. But they should have the opportunity to make an informed choice, and, most importantly, be at peace with that choice.'

Other factors that can increase your risk of breast cancer

Every day we make decisions that involve weighing up risks and benefits. Deciding whether or not to take HRT should be no different.

If you're worried about the risk of HRT because you've had breast cancer, it's important to look at other areas of your life that increase your risk and how you can address these, too, so that if you do decide to proceed with HRT, you are minimising your overall risk as much as possible.

The lifestyle factors that can increase your risk of breast cancer are: being very overweight (BMI of 30 or more), drinking alcohol most days, smoking and a lack of physical exercise.

Family history of breast cancer

Most women will have a history of breast cancer in their family because it is a relatively common disease. Family history includes any 'first-degree' relatives, including your mother, father, brothers, sisters and any children you may have, and 'second-degree' relatives, including aunts, uncles, grandparents, nieces and nephews.

Researchers estimate that only around 5–10 per cent of breast cancers are caused by an inherited faulty gene.[171]

A lot of women have their ovaries removed because there is also an increased risk of cancer of the ovaries in some who have a family history of breast cancer. After this operation, they will become menopausal. Others will become menopausal for different reasons, usually due to age.

If you have a family history of breast cancer, you may be wondering what your options are regarding treatment, particularly HRT.

There is no strong evidence that a family history of breast cancer puts you at any higher risk of getting the disease if you take HRT, compared to women who do not have a family history.[172]

There is some evidence that women with a family history of breast cancer who take HRT actually have a lower future risk of developing it compared to those with a family history of breast cancer who do not take it.[173]

This means that women with a family history of breast cancer, including those with a BRCA gene, can still usually take HRT safely. Many choose to take it for its future health benefits.

Menopause after a cancer diagnosis: making decisions about treatment with your doctor or other healthcare professional

Guidelines from the General Medical Council and recommendations from NICE show how decisions should be made between a patient and doctor and specify that a shared decision-making process should take place, involving the following:[174, 175]

- The patient should be encouraged to take an active role in making decisions about their treatment, considering what is most important to them, their expressed needs and their priorities. Treatment options should be explained in light of these factors.
- Open discussion of the risks, benefits and consequences of each treatment option (including doing nothing), with the acceptance that the patient's views can differ from the professionals'.

- Enough time to answer questions and make decisions, making it clear that the patient can change their mind down the line.
- A joint decision that is satisfactory to the patient.

All patients have the right to be adequately informed about and involved in decisions about their treatment. This means the information that healthcare professionals give about HRT should be based on the best available evidence when discussing the associated risks and benefits. This should include information about the various ways to take HRT and an explanation of how any risks are particularly relevant to *you*.

Here are some tips to help you in your discussions with your doctor:

- Do your own research and be prepared.
- Keep a record of your symptoms to show a clear account of their range and severity and how they're affecting your daily life. You could use the free balance menopause support app to do this or complete the menopause symptom questionnaire (see Resources, p. 360). You can also use these tools to measure any improvement in your symptoms once you start treatment.
- If you're considering systemic HRT or vaginal hormones, learn about the options and think about which type you might prefer.
- Plan the time you need to discuss matters adequately – you might want to ask for a double slot or spread discussions out over separate appointments.
- Write comments or questions down if you're worried about forgetting in the moment.

- Inform your doctor in advance about what you want to discuss; this will ensure that you get the most out of your consultation and will give them the opportunity to do their own research, too. It will also allow them time to discuss your case with local specialists, find out about the most appropriate specialist clinics or direct you to someone in the practice who has an interest in the topic.

- Be persistent but polite. If you do not get the desired outcome at the first appointment, you have a right to ask for a second opinion. You can ask to see another clinician within your practice. Ask which member of the team has an interest in menopause or women's health or whether there is an NHS menopause specialist clinic in your area. Another option is to book an appointment with a private menopause specialist.

Find support

The experience of going through cancer treatments and then finding out you're in the menopause can feel very isolating and may make you want to withdraw from friends and family and try to deal with things on your own. Although this is a very normal reaction, after a while it can often lead to you feeling like everything is getting on top of you, and you might struggle to cope.

Find a family member or friend who is a good listener, doesn't judge you, makes you feel safe and gives you the time and space to talk about how you're feeling. If you don't have someone like this, counselling can be really helpful. You can ask for this via your GP or find a professional yourself online (see Resources, p. 359). As well as thinking about one-to-one counselling, being part of a network of people who have been through something similar can help to reduce feelings of isolation and fear and provide a space that is supportive. There are many charities with online chat forums and support groups for people going through cancer (see Resources).

It is important to know that any decision you make about treatment is reversible, and you can change your mind at any time. It is essential that you feel in control of all decision making.

9

Unseen and Unheard: Why the Menopause Conversation Must Be More Inclusive

What you will learn in this chapter:

1. Why we have to dispel the myth that menopause is only relevant to White, heterosexual, middle-class women

2. Research highlighting disparities in menopause care

3. About the people helping to make menopause more inclusive

4. Tips on how to transform the conversation in your own community

Preparing recently for my PowerPoint slides for a lecture at the International Menopause Society conference entitled 'Ethnic disparities in UK menopause care', I was looking for some picture inspiration. I ran a search for 'menopausal woman' into the images section of a search engine and, in under a second, my screen was filled with all the usual menopause clichés. Stock photoshoot pictures of a woman perched on the end of a sofa or bed, a hand to her forehead, or head in hands; a woman puffing out her cheeks while fanning herself with a hand-held fan; a woman gazing into the middle distance or out of a window in her neutrally decorated home . . .

All the models were White, all were middle-aged, and all were wearing reassuringly expensive clothing (some even sporting a respectable string of pearls). It took a fair bit of scrolling down to find a woman of colour. And I gave up before I was able to find a picture of someone who looked like they were under the age of forty.

The results were completely at odds with the wording of my presentation, which was all about how menopause affects half of society, regardless of background, socioeconomic status or orientation.

I snapped my laptop shut, feeling frustrated. But a few minutes later, I went back to the same page and took a screenshot to use in my presentation.

Why? Because that one search summed up the entire problem with the menopause image and, as such, it perfectly backed up the content of my presentation.

While the menopause itself doesn't discriminate, the conversation *around* it does. The perimenopause and menopause certainly does not just affect White, married, heterosexual women. It happens to all of us, whether Black, White, Asian, heterosexual, lesbian, gay or trans. Menopause also affects those living with long-term conditions, those struggling with addiction, those living in poverty, those in prison.

This chapter shines a spotlight on unrepresented groups, looking to the future as to how we, as a society, can make the menopause conversation as inclusive as it should be, as well as providing advice on how you can advocate for yourself.

What do we know about racial differences in the perimenopause and menopause?

It'll probably come as no surprise that amid a lack of research into women's health in general, there isn't an abundance of research into diverse experiences of menopause. But of the research that *has* been carried out, much of it in the United States, there are some themes.

Menopause can occur earlier if you are from a non-White background. A 2022 study found that Black women have their final period an average of eight and a half months before White women.[176] According to the analysis, Black women were 50 per cent more likely than White women to report hot flushes, while 27 per cent of Black women reported clinically significant depressive symptoms, compared to 22 per cent of White women.

In addition, preliminary research found that Black women were three times more likely to become menopausal before the age of forty.[177] In the analysis, involving 3,522 Black women and 6,514 White women, menopause at a young age occurred in 15.5 per cent of Black women and 4.8 per cent of White women.

Research shows that women from South Asian backgrounds tend to become menopausal earlier, at around forty-six years of age. Several studies have indicated that women living in developing countries (including Latin America, Indonesia, Singapore,

Pakistan, Chile and Peru) experience natural menopause several years earlier than those in developed countries. It is unclear whether these geographic and international differences reflect genetic, socioeconomic, environmental, racial/ethnic or lifestyle differences.[178]

Some studies also that show women in different countries experience the menopause with different symptoms.[179] Women from South Asian backgrounds whose diets may be more plant based (containing phytoestrogens, which can stimulate the oestrogen receptors) tend to suffer from fewer hot flushes, night sweats and skin changes.[180] However, these women commonly have more body aches, palpitations and urinary symptoms. In addition, women from South Asian backgrounds have a higher risk of cardiovascular disease, type 2 diabetes, insulin resistance, obesity and osteoporosis than the White population.[181] When they are menopausal, these risks increase further.

Menopausal women from all ethnicities will have low hormone levels, regardless of which symptoms they are experiencing – or even if they are not experiencing symptoms.

SURVEY: RACIAL DISPARITIES IN MENOPAUSE CARE

Almost 14 per cent of the UK population is from a minority-ethnic background – and in London, this rises to 40 per cent.[182] Yet swathes of society from minority backgrounds are being left out of the menopause conversation, not only in the media, but in the consulting room, too.

Let me share some data. Last year, my team and I worked with the journalist, author, producer and menopause activist Kate

Muir to analyse the results of a large-scale survey into meno-pause in the UK (we will be hearing from Kate on p. 353).[183] The original online survey was carried out on behalf of the Fawcett Society, a charity that campaigns for gender equality and women's rights. It was open to women aged forty-five to fifty-five with current menopausal symptoms and had 4,014 respondents.

The data was weighted, so it would to be representative of UK women. Women from Black British and Asian backgrounds made up 8 per cent of the respondents, which is largely consistent with women in this age group in the UK – about 7.5 per cent of the UK population are from an Asian background, including Indian, Pakistani, Bangladeshi and Chinese.[184]

The findings make for uncomfortable reading. Strikingly, there were several significant differences between menopause care for White women and those from non-White backgrounds.

While there were no ethnic differences in terms of symptoms, White British women were twice as likely to be receiving HRT for their symptoms compared to Black British and British Asian women (15 per cent for White women, compared to 8 per cent for women with a non-White/ethnic-minority background). We also found that non-White women were 38 per cent more likely to be hesitant about taking HRT due to perceived risks, and 50 per cent more likely to say they had experienced barriers to menopause care.

Half (54 per cent) of non-White respondents reported low levels of motivation.

In this day and age, these findings are shameful and under-score the fact that while in general the menopause conversation is changing for the better, it's not getting better for everyone.

Fortunately, there are many groups aiming to support these discussions, such as People Arise Now, a charitable organisation. Their goal is to change the dialogue and challenge the taboo by talking about the menopause within these communities. They are breaking down the barriers to support women and men in asking the questions that need answers. Dr Claire Phipps, one of the doctors who works closely with me in my clinic, spoke at one of their events in 2022. She explained:

> It was a privilege to be invited to hold space with these women and to be able to talk about what the perimenopause and menopause meant to them and their communities. We shared our personal journeys and broke down a lot of myths about this time. We also all agreed how more education of our health professionals is needed and how we can strive to make the perimenopause and menopause a positive transition; provided the right information is being delivered.

Reframing conversations to break down cultural barriers

Research published in 2022 found that British women are more comfortable talking about their menopause.[185]

On the surface, that sounds like a really positive finding. But when you look at the overall results of this survey, which asked women from thirty-three countries for their views on menopause, it found that women globally were happier to talk about their age, physical health, ethnicity, religion and mental health than they were about their menopause.

Or, putting it another way, women are often more comfortable about talking about anything *but* their menopause. So how can we redress this?

Healthcare professionals can play a huge part in paving the way for more meaningful conversations. And those conversations need to take into account cultural differences. Firstly, they need to be aware that these may affect the way women report their symptoms. As Meera explains (her story is shared in this chapter), there isn't even a word for menopause in some languages.

And we have to be sensitive to the nuances of what the menopause means to women in different cultures. For some, because the menopause means the end of periods it can feel like quite a liberating moment in their lives. I've spoken to women who have been living with HIV for decades for whom menopause is a cause for celebration, because it was a life milestone they didn't think they would live to see. For some religious faiths, not having a period is again liberating as they are allowed to pray and attend their places of worship more frequently.

But for others, especially those who are religious and also young, the end of menstruation marks the end of their fertility and that can be difficult to come to terms with.

Why we need tailored information

Better care starts with conversations. And those conversations need more tailored information.

But how many GP surgeries and websites (including the NHS website) provide adequate menopause resources in English, let alone in other languages?

We have to make information more accessible to the communities we work in, including providing interpreters where needed.

At balance, my menopause app, we've worked hard to make sure our resources are as accessible as possible. This has included translating some of our most-read resources into Hindi, Chinese, Welsh, French and Spanish, with the help of volunteers including Dr Radhika Vohra, Dr Laurena Law and Dr Brigitte Letombe.

We have also produced information posters in a range of languages, and have translated a course on creating a menopause-confident organisation into eleven languages.

EXPERT VIEW
Why we created a menopause group for women of colour – Dr Martina Toby and Dr Nneka Nwokolo

Dr Martina and Dr Nneka are consultant physicians in sexual health and HIV medicine, with a special interest in menopause. They joined forces to help educate and advocate for women of colour experiencing perimenopause and menopause through the @shadesofmenopause Instagram group. Here, they explain why they set up their group.

For us, menopause is one of the most rewarding aspects of medicine. For some women, menopause symptoms make their lives almost unlivable, but, with guidance and treatment, we can help them get back to living their lives, enjoying their work and their families.

In 2020, we were jointly invited to host a forum about menopause for women of colour. Dozens of women joined the forum and, as we listened to them sharing their stories, the prevailing theme was that they didn't feel seen or listened to.

So many women who attended the forum said they felt grateful, not only to find out more about the menopause from specialists of colour, but also for the opportunity to speak openly about their experiences.

One woman even started to cry: she told us she had never felt able to speak out about the impact of menopause and what she was going through until that moment. For us, that forum was a catalyst – we knew then that we had to do something to reach more women, and that's when the initial idea for our Instagram group, Shades of Menopause, was born.

Shades of Menopause is a place where all women can come for perimenopause and menopause information, with everything from symptoms to treatments to busting menopause myths.

We wanted it to be a place where women of colour could ask questions, share their own stories and offer advice to their peers, and it is going from strength to strength. Because it is run by healthcare professionals, women know it is valid and evidence based. That is particularly reassuring for women of colour, who can be sceptical about the healthcare system.

If you are a woman on your own perimenopause and menopause journey, our three key pieces of advice would be as follows:

1. Do your own research and ask other women about their experiences.

2. See your GP for help. Ask who is the best person to see at your practice. Go equipped with knowledge already, and you will get a much better outcome.

3. Remember you are not alone – millions of women like you are going through it. If you feel you can't speak up, find a friend who is willing to do it for you. Your voice matters and needs to be heard.

CASE STUDY: SPEAKING OUT ABOUT
MENOPAUSE IN MY COMMUNITY
AND AT WORK – MEERA'S STORY

When Meera started to develop symptoms of menopause at the age of forty, she didn't know where to turn for advice. She's since implemented free menopause training to support women in the workplace and is committed to bringing menopause into the open in South Asian communities.

'In South Asian culture there's no word for "menopause", and, for many, female health is very much a taboo subject. So when I tried to talk to my mother about the new symptoms I was experiencing, she dismissed my concerns. Even though I had only just turned forty, my hair was thinning, my skin was changing, my periods were debilitating and erratic, my joints ached and I lacked energy. I didn't recognise myself at all, as I'd always been super active, busy and living life to the fullest. I found that I was no longer able to do things that were normal for me, and I was losing my confidence.

'I spoke to my GP, who said I was too young for the menopause and offered me antidepressants. I didn't know where to turn.

'In the end, it was my yoga teacher who linked my symptoms to menopause. So I went on a mission to learn more, and used my new-found knowledge to change my diet and lifestyle. I learned that my risk of osteoporosis was increasing, so I started doing resistance training, and I focused on eating the foods that were most beneficial to me. I also developed a love for weight training. As a result, I'm now stronger, fitter, healthier and leaner than I was in my twenties and thirties.

'After everything I went through, I'm passionate about opening up the conversation about menopause, particularly in South Asian communities where it's just not spoken about. I've implemented free

HR training on menopause at the nursery I run, and I've also developed other staff initiatives, such as appointing a menopause champion, offering flexible and home working for those experiencing perimenopause and menopause and providing wellness baskets in the bathrooms (containing things like sanitary products and deodorants).

'I think it's so important to champion menopause warriors in the workplace and ensure that there's a supportive and inclusive atmosphere. If all businesses could implement menopause training, I believe that staff would be better placed to support their co-workers and help more women to have a positive experience of menopause.'

We need to anticipate different questions

A wake-up call for me came a few years ago during a patient consultation.

My patient was a Black woman, who was outwardly very successful with a strong and happy marriage, but she had become a shell of her former self, as she struggled with worsening migraines during the perimenopause.

During the consultation, we discussed her symptoms, and it became apparent that she would benefit from HRT. I talked her through the different methods, and how patches and gels were particularly suited to women with migraines, due to the reduced risk of clots.

As someone who also suffers from migraines, I felt like I was on familiar ground and could relate to her experiences. But as I talked through the options, I could sense my patient seemed to be very resistant to the idea of patches. I knew it wasn't a reticence to take HRT per se, as my patient had said she wanted to try it at the outset.

After talking more, it emerged that she was very concerned as to whether patches were suitable for darker skin tones and wanted to know what evidence I had.

While there is no biological reason why absorption through darker skin would be any different to that through lighter skin – and I tried to reassure her to that effect – that conversation taught me a valuable lesson. I felt at a loss because I didn't have the right language and I didn't have the research she was looking for, because, as a White doctor, it was question I hadn't even considered in enough detail before.

After some discussion, my patient decided to try patches, and I'm pleased to say she saw an improvement in her symptoms. But for me, the encounter made me conscious of the fact that she deserved a more individualised conversation.

As healthcare professionals, we need to put ourselves in our patients' shoes. We need to be aware of different health and cultural beliefs and, if unsure, ask the patient what *they* want to know.

Perimenopause and menopause in LGBTQ+ communities

It's a sad fact that members of the LGBTQ+ community all too often feel excluded from healthcare services in general.

Research shows that one in eight LGBT people (13 per cent) in Britain has experienced some form of unequal treatment from healthcare staff because they're LGBT, while one in four (23 per cent) has witnessed discriminatory or negative remarks against LGBT people by healthcare staff.[186] One in seven LGBT people (14 per cent) has avoided treatment for fear of discrimination because they're LGBT.[187]

And when it comes to menopause, the LGBTQ+ community can be even more isolated. Research around LGBTQ+ experiences is lacking, and online resources are scant.

And even if you do get through the door of your local GP surgery or clinic, the discussion isn't always relevant. Advice about partners often assumes women are in heterosexual relationships and any contraception advice is centred around prevention of pregnancy – not exactly relevant for those in same-sex relationships.

I have many patients who are in same-sex relationships and some women have told me that the conversation with other healthcare professionals about the menopause has only focused on fertility rather than on menopausal symptoms.

One young patient with POI who is in her mid-twenties was actually told by her gynaecologist that she 'need not worry about the menopause and fertility, as there are two wombs in her relationship', looking over at her female partner who had come along to support her. Understandably, she left the consultation very upset and then did not have the confidence to seek help and treatment for her menopause until she was a few years older.

The conversation gets even more challenging if you are a transgender man. Any trans or nonbinary person who was assigned female at birth but who hasn't undergone any medical interventions, such as masculinising HRT or hysterectomy, is likely to go through menopause eventually. Trans men and non-binary people assigned female at birth may experience menopause if they keep their ovaries and do not alter their hormone doses with time.

However, because they are often not represented in the language around healthcare, they risk losing access to individualised menopause care entirely.

For trans women taking oestrogen, there is no need to stop this treatment at any particular age or after taking it for a specific length of time, in the same way that others do not need to stop taking HRT at a certain age.

At the time of writing, NICE is reviewing its guidelines for healthcare professionals on menopause, and has already indicated that the next version will be more inclusive. For the first time, NICE says the updated document explicitly includes trans and non-binary people, alongside cisgender women.

This is a big step forward and couldn't come sooner.

Timeout #1: How to make your menopause-related appointment tailored to you

If you have an appointment coming up, here are a few steps to ensure the conversation is individualised to you.

- Think about your symptoms: have you logged them to bring to the appointment?
- Do you have a long-term condition or specific risk factors for other diseases like diabetes? Ask how menopause may impact this.
- Are there any local support groups that you might benefit from?

Menopause in marginalised communities

....

For many people living with long-term conditions, or in marginalised communities, they can be defined by their condition or status.

Menopause can be overlooked, meaning that many women are not seeking the right help, advice and treatment. If they do try, many of them are misdiagnosed or given incorrect treatment. Too often, I have heard from women that they have not been believed when they have tried to explain the nature and variety of their symptoms. All women deserve to be listened to and understood.

Menopause and HIV

In 2019, I was at a British Menopause Society conference and heard a lecture from Dr Shema Tariq presenting results of the PRIME study. This is one of the largest studies globally looking at the impact of the menopause on the health and wellbeing of women living with HIV, with data on nearly 900 women aged forty-five to sixty.[188]

I learned that women living with HIV are more likely to suffer with menopausal symptoms and less likely to receive HRT, which I was really surprised and saddened to hear. When I asked Dr Tariq afterwards why clinicians running HIV clinics do not prescribe HRT, she explained that they have no menopause training and they often don't know how to prescribe it.

I thought about what I could do to change this, and contacted an organisation called the Sophia Forum, which works with women living with HIV, offering to work with them to develop a booklet about the menopause.

Menopause and female genital mutilation (FGM)

More than 200 million girls and women alive today have under-gone female genital mutilation, a human-rights violation that involves the partial or total removal of external female genitalia or other injury to the female genital organs for non-medical reasons.

It can cause severe bleeding and problems urinating, cysts, infections, complications in childbirth and increased risk of newborn deaths.

FGM is typically performed on young girls and adolescents in some regions of Africa, the Middle East and Asia, and in communities around the world originating from these areas, including in the UK.

Reasons vary, but it is usually carried out in response to social pressures, conforming to cultural ideals of femininity and modesty, virginity and fidelity.[189]

In the UK, it is estimated that some 137,000 women have undergone FGM and some 60,000 girls under fifteen years old are at risk.[190] And every one of them will become menopausal and may require specialist care.

The majority of menopausal women will experience symptoms related to genitourinary syndrome of the menopause; women who have been cut are more likely to have more severe symptoms, as the tissues in the vaginal and vulval area are already scarred and thinner compared to other women. It is essential that these women have access to treatment as replacing hormones in these tissues is likely to really improve their local-ised symptoms.

However, there have shockingly been no studies undertaken on menopausal urogenital health in women who have undergone female genital mutilation, and their needs are currently unaddressed.[191] This urgently needs to change.

In 2022, I met an incredible woman called Sarian Karim, who experienced FGM as a child in Sierra Leone. She founded grassroots organisation Keep the Drums Lose the Knife and works with communities and survivors to end FGM in Sierra Leone and the UK.

Inspiration can be an overused word, but Sarian is the embodiment of it, breaking down barriers, educating women and healthcare professionals and helping women to live healthier lives.

As this book goes to press, we are working together on a project to bring menopause education to FGM survivors in the UK.

Menopause in prisons

In 2000, when I was a newly qualified GP, I did a week's work in HMP Styal, a prison and young-offender institution for women in Cheshire, as their medical doctor. It was the hardest and most harrowing week's work I have ever done and a period I have reflected on so much over the past twenty or so years.

Many of the women were so young and had various psychiatric conditions, such as bipolar disorder, schizophrenia and clinical depression. Some of them had actually been born at Styal – there was a mother-and-baby unit there – and others were pregnant while serving their sentences.

For some, coming to the prison was a time when they were given attention, care and proper food. They were all friendly and respectful to me; many told me horrendous stories about their childhoods and the abuse they endured, both physical and emotional.

The medication that some of the women were taking for psychiatric disorders was actually suppressing their levels of follicule-stimulating hormone (FSH – as we saw earlier, a hormone produced in our brains that works to regulate oestrdaiol and testosterone levels). When FSH levels are low, then levels of oestradiol and testosterone are also reduced. This means that these medications can lead to a so-called 'chemical menopause'. I do often wonder how differently some of these women would have felt if they'd had these hormones replaced.

The women who were malnourished, those who were addicted to drugs and those who were alcoholics were very unlikely to be having regular periods. Yet never once did I think, as a health-care professional, about asking them about their periods.

In 2021, I wrote a newsletter all about the menopause and treatments available, which went to all prisons in the UK, but I have always wanted to do more. In 2022, this became a reality when the balance app team began a perimenopause-and-meno-pause-education programme in prisons for women and prison staff, including healthcare professionals working in prisons.

Menopause and domestic abuse

There is growing evidence that domestic violence can increase during the perimenopause and menopause. This domestic abuse can be physical or emotional, or both.[192]

Many women have told me that they feel so utterly dreadful and lack so much confidence that they 'deserve' to be abused, as they are not the people they should be. Others have openly admitted that they have shouted without good reason at their children or loved ones, as they have felt so short-tempered and irritable.

Menopause and addiction and eating disorders

Many people do not realise that addictive behaviours can increase during the perimenopause and menopause – this is thought to be due to the powerful effect of the loss of sex hormones on the brain. Drinking more alcohol, taking drugs, gambling, eating disorders and gaming are all behaviours that can escalate and become out of control when hormone levels are low.[193]

Finding your voice – and using it to transform the conversation

If you are struggling with menopause symptoms and are feeling isolated because of who you are, I want you to know that you are not alone. There are incredible healthcare professionals, campaign groups and lone activists who are working behind the scenes to ensure everyone feels part of the menopause conversation.

Here are some tips on how to make your voice heard.

Already under the care of a healthcare team? Ask if you need specialist menopause care

You may already be under the care of a team due to a long-term problem, such as a mental-health condition, diabetes or hypertension, which means that you will be seeing healthcare professionals regularly. Some of these may have had training in the perimenopause and menopause. But if you feel that you might benefit from more specialist menopause care, you can ask for a referral.

Turn to your peer networks

Friends and family can be a place to share experiences of menopause (if they are perimenopausal or menopausal, you may find they too are looking for someone to talk to), and they can be a source of support if you feel nervous about attending appointments. You can also ask your healthcare professional to signpost any local face-to-face support groups that might help you.

Social media can help

If you don't have a close group of friends or feel like you can talk to family, then look further afield for other supportive spaces where you have access to the right information. I'll be completely honest: I originally set up my own Instagram page purely to keep an eye on what my teenage daughters were up to, but over the years it has grown into the most incredible, informative and supportive network for lots of people. It was my daughters who schooled me in the ways of Instagram and showed me how important posting every day is to keep you engaged with your followers. It's a great place to share short videos, soundbites and treatment updates and impart my knowledge in a way that is completely free, open and accessible.

Instagram is my social network of choice. However, there are of course other social media channels you can try. You might prefer the more rapid, quick-fire nature of Twitter, Facebook for closed groups or even LinkedIn, if you want to connect with others doing things to spread menopause awareness in the workplace. And don't forget TikTok: my friend and GP Dr Nighat Arif has used TikTok videos to great effect in communicating key menopause messages, particularly to South Asian communities.

In addition, the balance app has a community area where people share stories and experiences. So many others have commented on these posts and they have really helped so many women in this way.

Bring others with you

Don't keep your new-found menopause knowledge to yourself! Use it to help others. You could share this book, or other resources, such as leaflets, podcasts or social media accounts you've found helpful.

Or take it a step further; be like Meera and get out there and talk about your own experiences in your community and beyond.

The more we talk about menopause, the better.

10

Why Exercise Is One of the Best Forms of Medicine

Four things you will learn in this chapter:

1. Why exercise is essential during the perimenopause and menopause

2. Why exercise is to be enjoyed, not endured

3 How to form an exercise habit – and stick with it

4. The best activities for healthy bones, heart and weight

Too hot. Too cold. Too tired. Too embarrassed. Don't have the right kit . . .

It sounds like the litany of excuses one of my daughters would come up with to duck out of a school sports lesson. But how many times in the past year have you used one of the above to convince yourself you don't need to exercise?

I'm what I would call active, rather than superfit, and I definitely didn't inherit sporty genes. Running cross country at school on damp winter mornings was my idea of absolute hell. By the time I was at medical school in the 1980s, step aerobics was all the rage; it might have been more energetic and, unlike running, had the bonus of being an indoor activity, but I absolutely hated that, too.

Swimming? I really enjoyed that as a student, but the whole palaver of washing my hair to get all the chlorine out and getting changed in damp-smelling changing rooms before rushing back to lectures was enough to make me retire my swimming goggles for good.

From boxercise to body pump, I dabbled with many other forms of exercise over the years but never seemed to find my comfort zone. Then, nineteen years ago, I went to my first Ashtanga yoga class. Ashtanga is a dynamic form of yoga where the same poses or 'postures' are performed in the same sequence, whether you do it alone or guided by a teacher in a group setting.

I remember tiptoeing into my first class, marvelling at the various positions other class members could mould their bodies into. I just thought, There's no way I can do this; and, if I'm honest, I really wanted to run for the hills. But I stayed for the practice, went back the following week and slowly but surely built up my stamina and strength over the years to the point where yoga has become an indispensable part of my physical and mental toolkit.

When I was perimenopausal but hadn't yet realised it, not even my beloved yoga could get me out of my rut. Like any physical activity, you have to keep doing it to see the benefits, but my joints were stiff and my muscles were sore. If you do yoga yourself, you'll know that if you have a really good practice, everything flows really well and you get a wonderful buzz and renewed sense of energy. Only, back then, I'd finish my practice feeling stiff, rusty and old.

I was tired, fed up and had no desire to exercise, so I stopped. And as the weeks went by, I could see the muscle tone I'd built up over a decade was starting to disappear before my very eyes.

Thankfully, my impetus for exercise returned once I started taking HRT, but those months where not even yoga appealed have always been a real lesson to me in how easily and how quickly we can get out of the habit of exercise.

With this in mind, whether you are a lapsed exerciser looking for ways to get active again or you have never found an activity to suit you, this chapter is all about forming some new habits to keep you happy and healthy from your perimenopause through to your post-menopause years.

Why exercise is a gateway to better health and wellbeing

I've faced a lot of criticism at times from those who say I 'medicalise' the menopause, as though I offer up HRT as the panacea for all. While I do – and will continue to – raise awareness about the benefits of HRT (and for the vast majority of women those benefits far outweigh the risks), HRT is just one part of the story. Because whether or not you decide to take it, you should still be keeping an eye on your current and future health beyond HRT alone. For example, if you take HRT but then rely on processed foods, don't exercise, drink alcohol to excess, smoke or have bad sleep habits, you are setting yourself up for poor health. So you need to take a 360-degree look at your life and think to yourself, Am I doing what I can to ensure I have a healthy future?

A simple, cost-effective way (and potentially free, depending on where and how you do it) to improve your overall health and wellbeing is through exercise. Along with actions like quitting smoking, physical activity is what is known as a modifiable risk factor against disease – because you *can* do something about it.

From building strength to protecting our brains, let's look at the multitude of benefits being physically active can bring.

Good for your heart

A 2022 survey of 8,000 UK adults found that women are more likely to report barriers to exercise than men, with more than half citing lack of motivation (67 per cent) and lack of time (55 per cent) as the main causes.[194]

A 2015 study found that middle-aged women could significantly lower their risk of heart disease and stroke by exercising just two to three times a week.[195] Researchers found women who did strenuous physical activity that was enough to cause sweating or a fast heartbeat two to three times a week, or any activity four to six times a week, had a 20 per cent lower risk of coronary heart disease, stroke and blood clots, compared to women who were inactive. And compared to being inactive, doing any form of physical activity (including walking, gardening and cycling) at least once a week was found to lower the risk of heart disease.

A 2020 study from the US-based National Cancer Institute and the National Institute on Aging found that higher daily step counts were associated with lower mortality risk from all causes, including cardiovascular disease.[196]

Meanwhile, a separate study found that exercise lowers the risk of repeat hospital admissions and mortality in women with coronary artery disease, as well as reducing stress and risk of hypertension and obesity.[197]

Reduced risk of dementia

According to the charity Alzheimer's UK, of all the lifestyle changes that have been studied, taking regular physical exercise appears to be one of the best things you can do to reduce your risk of getting dementia.[198] It says studies looking at aerobic exercise (exercise that increases your heart rate) in middle-aged or older women and men have reported improvements in thinking and memory, and reduced rates of dementia.

Bone protection

Several studies have shown that weight-bearing exercise can help to slow bone loss and may even help to build bone.[199, 200]

Combats menopausal weight gain

When you build muscle through exercise, it helps your body to burn calories more efficiently, which, in turn, helps to shed any excess weight. It's important to point out that exercise alone won't result in weight loss so, if you are looking to lose a few pounds, you need to consider your diet, too – the nutrition chapter in this book has a section looking at weight loss (see pp. 302–04).

Aids restful sleep

You might be reading this on the back of another bad night's sleep thanks to night sweats, anxiety or needing to get up in the night to use the toilet. Exercise might seem like the last thing you want to do but exerting yourself in this way during the day helps set you up for a good night's sleep, studies having shown that regular exercise does indeed have a positive impact on sleep quality and duration.[201, 202]

Plus, if you exercise outside (going for a walk or a run, say), exposing yourself to daylight can help to regulate your body's wake–sleep cycle.

Aids digestion

Physical activity can increase the blood flow to the muscles in your digestive system that move food along the digestive tract.

Timeout #1: When was the last time you enjoyed exercise?

Take a few minutes to think about the last time you exercised.

- What was it about the exercise that you enjoyed? Was it the pace, the location, the people?
- And if you didn't enjoy it, why not? Was the gym too crowded? A home workout too solitary? Was the exercise itself too hard or too slow?
- Think of three things you want to get out of exercise: for example, getting out of the house, losing weight, meeting new people, taking some time for yourself?

Starting out

In my experience, the women who have the best menopause are those who take a holistic approach to their health. And central to that is exercise. But it is hard to feel motivated when your knees hurt, you've put on weight or you're worried about having a hot flush in the middle of a workout.

The best advice I can give is to start small and work your way up to a regular exercise routine. The UK government guidelines for exercise state that adult women should be exercising for half an hour a day, five times a week, as well as doing strength exercises on two days a week.[203]

When it's written down like that, it seems like an awful lot. However, if you stop thinking about 'exercise' and start thinking about 'activity' instead, it suddenly feels a lot more manageable. And you don't have to be in full workout gear or inside a gym or dance studio to do it. A brisk walk to the bus stop in the morning on the way to work, and the same again in the evening? Playing chase with your children or grandchildren in the park? Doing a spot of weeding? All this counts towards your weekly exercise targets.

EXPERT VIEW
Yoga 101 – Lucy Holtom,
Perimenopause and menopause teacher

Perimenopause and menopause teacher Lucy Holtom has been practising yoga for nearly thirty years and works alongside me at my clinic, and on my balance app.

Yoga can be a great support during your perimenopause and menopause journey, giving you coping tools and helping you feel grounded as you navigate this period of change. It is a practice that encapsulates a series of movements, known as poses or postures, breathing, meditation and relaxation, and it teaches us that any impact on the body will affect the mind, and vice versa, and that the breath is key in making us feel at ease.

I first discovered yoga as a teenager and taught myself some basic poses using a 1970s Vogue book, before attending my first yoga class aged nineteen. I can remember that first class like it was yesterday: it was led by a woman in her sixties, and I felt totally inspired by her teaching. From experiencing a sense of class unity in making shapes with our bodies, to the practice of meditation and discovering how to breathe with the whole body, I was totally hooked, and it set me on a path for my life's work.

How can yoga help you through the perimenopause and menopause?

Studies show the benefits of yoga for menopause symptoms, such as reducing insomnia and improvement in sleep quality.[204] A review paper investigating the effects of yoga on menopausal symptoms in thirteen randomised trials with a total of 1,300 participants found it helped to reduce psychological and urinogenital symptoms, and others, such as hot flushes and night sweats.[205]

Yoga is also beneficial for bone health. As Dr Louise has covered earlier in this book, bone density reduces as you get older, and yoga helps build bone strength through a series of weight-bearing movements. Stronger bones mean fewer fractures.

Other physical benefits include strengthening the pelvic floor and improving joint mobility and digestive health – all important areas that can be impacted by falling hormone levels.

As a teacher who regularly holds classes for perimenopausal and menopausal women, I've seen first-hand the positive impact regular practice can bring.

Any side effects?

Side effects from yoga are rare, but people can experience the usual aches and pains that come after any form of exercise. Be sure to let your yoga teacher know of any health issues, such as back problems or high blood pressure, as you may want to skip certain postures. And if you have concerns about the suitability of yoga for you, speak to your healthcare professional.

Getting started

Yoga can be practised alone in your own home using online or pre-recorded classes or, better still, in a class, chosen to suit your level and with guidance from a teacher.

If you do prefer to go it alone and are a beginner, just make sure you start slow and take your time.

Yoga is always practised barefoot, and you should opt for comfortable, breathable clothes that allow free movement – leggings and a sleeveless tank top are ideal.

And don't forget to use a yoga mat – this will help to improve your grip, support your joints and reduce the risk of injury from slipping.

Why there is no 'right' or 'wrong' exercise during perimenopause and menopause

Recent UK figures show that 35 per cent of people aged forty-five to fifty-four are not phsyically active, with men being more active than women.[206] At the very time women should be thinking about making changes to safeguard their future health, they are turning away from exercise. Why?

When I speak to perimenopausal and menopausal women who are inactive, or who have stopped exercising since becoming menopausal, their reasons are usually multifactorial. Physical symptoms are often a barrier, and self-esteem can play a part, too. But I also hear from a lot of women that they either view exercise as a chore or they fear they are doing it 'wrong'.

We all need to get out of the mindset that there is a right and a wrong way to exercise: just getting out there and moving your body is an achievement in itself and lays a foundation to build upon. So if a high-intensity internal training (HIIT) class hurts your knees, don't do it. Or maybe vaginal dryness means a spin class would be agony – again, don't do it.

Now I'm not going to give you a five-day menopause-busting workout plan that will see your joint pains and hot flushes disappear overnight. Your symptoms, overall fitness level and medical history will all be different to those of the next woman who picks up this book, so a one-size-fits-all approach just won't work.

When it comes to the type of exercise you do, I'm passionate about personal choice. Take my own exercise preferences, for example. I know the social aspect of exercise is a great added bonus and is important for lots of people but, for me, yoga suits my life because I'm in control of it. My job is incredibly hectic, and not having to head to a gym or a yoga studio to exercise or worry about missing a class if clinic runs late works for me. I can flick my yoga mat out any time, anywhere, whether at home early in the morning before work or in a hotel room, if I'm away at a conference.

Having said that, I'm incredibly lucky to have the best of both worlds, as I do have a yoga studio in my clinic where we run classes. Every Wednesday at 10am, I go to an ashtanga yoga class run by the inspirational James Critchlow, and everyone who works with me knows that time is sacred and is one of the rare times in a working week that people can't get hold of me on email.

The practice I do in the clinic studio is similar to the one I do at home on my own. James teaches three of us in the class and he is so calm and just a wonderful person to be around. While solo yoga is about making exercise work for me, the class is a great way to feel supported and motivated.

But whether at home or in my clinic, I don't see yoga as exercise; it's an activity that I love because it grounds me and keeps me strong – both physically and mentally. I know it won't be everyone's first choice, though – in the same way that a gym membership would be a waste of money for me, as I like the peace of exercising alone, in my own time and on my own terms.

So if you haven't found it already, you need to go out and find your yoga.

It can be confusing to know which exercise to go for, especially if it's been a while since you did any, so take advantage of free trials and taster classes; or ask a friend if they can get you a guest pass the next time they go to their gym.

If you live in England, the National Lottery-funded This Girl Can campaign (see Resources, p. 358) runs forty-five-minute classes specifically for those looking to get into exercise for the first time, or after a break. You'll try a different activity each week to give you a taster of various exercise-class styles (see Resources). If you live outside of England, try your local gym for a free taster session.

And if you don't like what you've tried, find something else. You wouldn't stick with an eight-season box set if you thought the first three episodes were too hard to follow or boring, would you? The same goes for activities. Don't feel obliged to carry on if you really can't stand them. There will be another exercise out there for you.

EXPERT VIEW
Exercise and perimenopause – Joe Wicks,
British fitness coach

Joe really needs no introduction. He kept the nation moving during the COVID-19 lockdowns, he's a fitness coach, a presenter, a bestselling author and an all-round fantastic person.

Joe and I first got talking in 2022, when he reached out to me as he wanted to know more about all things menopause, but particularly perimenopause. Since then, he has built up an incredible knowledge base, and I'm so pleased he's agreed to be a contributor to this book, providing advice on keeping active during the perimenopause and menopause.

I've been a qualified personal trainer now for just over ten years and, during that time, I have worked with hundreds of clients in person and helped hundreds of thousands of people with my online fitness plans and Body Coach App. I'm very passionate about helping people get stronger and healthier, and I work hard to promote the benefits of physical activity for our mental health.

But I have to be honest – I only very recently became aware of the term perimenopause. I had heard of the term menopause before but didn't know much about it. After receiving hundreds of messages on social media from women asking me for help and advice, I decided to do some research to gain a better understanding. What was the perimenopause? How did it affect body and mind? And how could I create workouts and recipes, and help, support, motivate and inspire women going through it?

That process has been such an eye opener for me. I've learned so much already and I have had some really great conversations. It has given me a much better understanding of the challenges women face when trying to stay active and strong during the perimenopause.

I've always been a big fan of and promoted high-intensity interval training (HIIT) for women for getting stronger and fitter. HIIT is a way of training that combines quick, intense bursts of exercise, where you're working out as hard as you can, with short periods of recovery. Getting your heart rate up to a level you can't sustain for long allows you to burn more fat in less time. HIIT is a great way of training, as it can be done with no equipment in a small space and in a short amount of time. This means it's an especially effective workout for those with a busy schedule and can get great results.

However, the more I learn about perimenopause and menopause, the more aware I am of the physical changes going on in the body, especially around the joints and with loss of lean muscle. So this type of high-impact exercise isn't always suitable for everyone. And if you are suffering from low energy levels and disrupted sleep, HIIT can be too intense and overwhelming.

While cardio exercise (the type of exercise that gets your heart rate up) is still great for the body and also for your mental health, rather than HIIT it may be better to focus on lower-impact, more gentle forms such as walking, cycling, cross training or rowing. This will allow you to get a good sweat on and improve your heart and lung health without the high impact on your joints.

Don't forget strength exercises

The best way to exercise is actually to focus on strength training. This could be done using slow, controlled body-weight moves, using dumbbells, resistance bands or even machines at the gym. With the focus on slower, controlled movements, and by increasing the resistance, you will be able to maintain and improve your strength and, with the right nutrition, build lean muscle.

It may feel like the last thing you want to do, but there is so much science now showing the link between physical movement and improved mental health. So with all the changes going on in your mind and body, it is the most powerful tool at your disposal. You will feel more energised, less stressed, calmer and happier after a workout. This may be a temporary boost but it's always worth it. You never regret a workout and will always feel better after.

Focus on the positives

Keep it simple and focus on the small daily wins. Listen to your body and don't be upset if you miss a workout or choose to take a nap instead. Be kind to yourself. Being sleep deprived makes everything feel hard, including moving and cooking and parenting. I've recently become a dad again and, when I get disturbed three or four times a night, I don't wake up energised and motivated in the morning. I wake up stressed and frustrated with stinging eyes. This is the reason I exercise daily. I use exercise to release those feelings. Exercise is something I need. And when you go through the peri-menopause, you need it, too – not just for fat loss and confidence, but for your mind and internal happiness.

Find the strength today to get moving, no matter how small or gentle the movements may be. All movement is positive and will help you get through difficult days.

Beneficial exercises for healthy heart, bones and mind

As I have covered, there is no 'wrong' exercise out there. The current guidelines talk about 'moderate' exercise, which essentially is something where you get out of puff, but you could still hold a conversation if you needed to.

Any form of movement that gets your heart rate up and blood pumping around your body is beneficial for your heart. The term aerobic literally means 'with oxygen' and describes exercises where your breathing and heart rate increase during the activity. Examples include brisk walking, swimming and aerobics.

When it comes to bone health, strength exercises are the ones to aim for. Here, you use your muscles to pull on your bones, which, in turn, makes them stronger. Yoga, Pilates and exercises using weights all count as strength exercises. In addition, weight-bearing exercises like walking and aerobics force your body to work against gravity, which helps to strengthen bones, too.

For mood and our minds, any type of physical exercise will release endorphins, which help to relieve pain and stress.

Building an exercise habit

You may not have any menopausal symptoms but still want to increase your exercise for future health. Or perhaps you have recently started HRT and want to harness the renewed energy and relief from symptoms.

Whatever your reasons, it pays to be sensible with your goals. Think about your baseline health: would it be more sensible to start with some gentle walks for the first week or two, or are you capable of something a bit more energetic?

Plan out when and where you want to exercise, being realistic about other work–life pressures, and write it down in your diary or set a reminder on your phone. One of the rare good things to come out of the COVID-19 pandemic was the realisation that we really can keep fit and healthy in the comfort of our own homes – so you could always keep close to home in the early days while you establish your routine.

And remember, self-care is not selfish. It's a fact of life that women are the gender who juggle the most. Research shows about 60 per cent of informal carers in the UK – someone who provides unpaid help to a friend or relative due to illness, age, disability or mental health condition – are women.[207] But while we all lead busy lives, it is vital you see exercise not as an optional extra, but as a core part of how you stay fit, healthy and happy. In the same way that you wouldn't view attending an important medical appointment or going to your dentist for a regular check-up as being selfish, exercise is part of the overall package.

CASE STUDY: EXERCISE WAS THE LAST THING I WANTED TO DO; BUT NOW I'VE GOT MY MOTIVATION BACK – LEAH'S STORY

Leah loved exercise and thought nothing of getting up at 6am and going for a run in the lanes near her home in the countryside. But when her menopause symptoms left her feeling flat and drained of energy, her love of exercise soon waned. Here, she describes how she got her motivation back – a great way to end this chapter.

'I struggled with my weight as a teenager and young adult. We were brought up never to leave anything on our plates. I had a huge appetite – I still do!

'I love chocolate and cakes and often overindulged and packed weight on easily. After putting on a lot of weight during my three pregnancies in my late twenties and early thirties, I joined a local Slimming World club and managed to lose three and a half stone in five months. Now I still eat lots, but it's the right kind of foods and I've maintained a healthy weight ever since.

'I really embraced exercise in my thirties, and my husband, three teenagers and I have a family membership for our local gym. Doing a workout or putting on my trainers and going for a run was part of my routine. I'm not one of those people who goes through the motions during exercise: I genuinely love it. When I exercise, I feel strong and fit and it helps to clear my head.

'A couple of years ago, in my forties, lots of little niggling symptoms started to creep up on me: I started picking up a few injuries and suffered with joint pain and stiffness. Having three teenagers and a busy job felt overwhelmingly emotional at times.

'Because of the aches and pains I couldn't exercise in the way I was used to, which was frustrating. I spent a lot of money on private physiotherapist appointments to try to get to the bottom of my aches and pains.

'I'm disciplined with food, so, while I never put on weight, I did lose my strength and tone.

'I'm really close to my two sisters and, after a conversation with my older sister, Anne, I came to the realisation that I was probably perimenopausal. I read up on the menopause and tried to work through it using the tools I had: nutrition and trying to exercise in different ways, such as lower impact exercise.

'But after a few months, I felt worse than ever and booked an appointment to see my GP. She was fantastic and really listened. I've now been on HRT for about eighteen months – the joint stiffness has gone.

'Most importantly, I can exercise the way I want to. I feel like I've got my mojo back, and I feel strong, healthy and happy – and I haven't been back to the physio since!'

SURVEY: OVERCOMING BARRIERS TO EXERCISE TO HELP YOU THRIVE DURING THE PERIMENOPAUSE AND MENOPAUSE

As we have covered throughout this chapter, the benefits of exercise during the perimenopause and menopause are numerous.

But my survey revealed that a lack of motivation is the biggest barrier to exercising at this time, followed by the impact of physical and psychological symptoms.

Walking was by far the most popular form of exercise, with 75 per cent of respondents saying it benefited their physical and mental health. Yoga, strength training and pilates were also popular.

11

Nutrition During the Perimenopause and Menopause

Four things you will learn in this chapter:

1. How what we eat can impact the perimenopause and menopause

2. The vitamins and minerals that can be beneficial through the menopause and beyond

3. Middle-aged spread: fact or fiction? And is it down to menopause?

4. How giving your gut some TLC can have a positive effect on your physical and mental wellbeing

You are what you eat, as the old adage goes. And while it might sound like a cliché, all in moderation is the mantra I tend to advise patients when it comes to food.

I eat healthily most of the time – because I know that if I don't, I soon start to feel sluggish and it can affect my moods. As a migraine sufferer, I also know that if I eat processed foods or foods high in sugar, I will develop a migraine, so avoiding these things is essential for me. I do not drink alcohol and I avoid caffeine (even in chocolate) – again to reduce the frequency of my migraines.

Of course, that doesn't mean I don't have the occasional treat. I am human, after all! My downfall is having a sweet tooth, but I have really 'trained' myself to avoid sugary foods as much as possible, and I can honestly say that I do not miss them now.

When I opened my clinic, I knew I wanted it to be about holistic care, looking at every aspect of our lives. And good food and nutrition form a huge part of the clinic, and this book too. But first, a few points on what this chapter *won't* be about.

It won't be advocating that you go on a 'diet': you won't find some super cleanse or other new-fangled eating plan to help you shift seven pounds in as many days. And it won't be about making you feel guilty for 'bad' food choices you have made thus far on your perimenopause and menopause journey.

What this chapter *will* do, however, is arm you with the knowledge and confidence needed to make small, sensible yet significant changes to the way you view food. Because I believe that the more we know about how to nourish our bodies, the more likely we are to make these changes. And that's why I have three fantastic experts on board.

Clinical nutritionist, chef and author Emma Ellice Flint has been working with me since the early days of my clinic. With a special interest in nutrition for women going through the perimenopause and menopause, she will be taking us through the twists and turns of how looking after our gut health can influ-ence how we feel.

A true food guru, Emma has incredible knowledge and is passionate about helping women to have the best possible peri-menopause and menopause. I knew I had to have her input when writing this book, and so I am thrilled she'll be sharing some of her knowledge here with you. Plus, as a former chef, Emma will also be sharing some recipes to help boost your mood, skin, gut and bone health; these are positively bursting with colour and flavour – and I should know, as I've been fortunate enough to have some lessons with Emma and have road tested a few of them myself.

We'll also be delving into why so many of us put on weight during menopause, and ways to tackle this. Providing expert advice will be Dr Sally Norton, a medical doctor, weight-loss consultant and the UK's first female weight-loss surgeon. If weight loss is part of your nutritional journey, her advice on why you need to set achievable, individual goals that aren't based on the latest diet fad will be invaluable.

And finally, we'll hear from Dr Rupy Aujla, an NHS medical doctor whose life was changed when he developed a significant heart condition. Dr Rupy started the fantastic Doctor's Kitchen blog and podcast as a way of teaching people how they can cook their way to health. He'll be looking at why food should be viewed as medicine, and has top tips for making healthy changes a permanent fixture on your plate.

Timeout #1: Is your diet the best it can be?

- Keep a three-day food diary. Write down everything you eat and drink. And that means *everything*. Had a couple of drinks, a few snacks or even finished off the leftovers from your child's plate? Write it all down.
- Think about how each meal makes you feel. Happy and satisfied? Or uncomfortable and bloated? Even a bit guilty?
- Have a peek in the fridge or look through your last supermarket shop receipt: are you really using everything you buy? What foods are regularly thrown away?
- Do a store-cupboard audit. So many of us will have packets and tins of staples hiding in the back of our cupboards that we've probably forgotten about. I know I've probably got enough packets of quinoa and rice to start my own restaurant. Before you look at making changes, save yourself money by checking what you already have to avoid duplication.

Finding balance in your diet

So now you know this chapter is not an exercise in finger-wagging, let's get started.

What have you eaten so far today? Was it homemade, served

up in a restaurant, canteen or coffee shop or did you purchase something on the run?

I'll start.

I'm writing this page on a Thursday evening.

Thursdays are dedicated clinic days for me, so that means an early start. Because I knew I had a long day ahead of me without a lot of time to spare, I ate my breakfast at 6.30am. This consisted of homemade granola, kefir (which I made myself from some grains that Emma gave me ages ago), Greek yoghurt and fresh fruit. It was tasty, visually appealing – thanks to the colour of the fruit – and I knew it would help to keep me full until my next meal.

I arrived at the clinic at 8am and patient consultations started at 9am.

Keeping hydrated is important and I only drink water or herbal teas (I carry herbal tea bags with me everywhere, so I know I can always have a hot drink when I am out).

I ate my lunch at 12.30pm while checking emails and preparing for the afternoon clinic. Because time is tight, I always bring something homemade with me. Today's lunch was a large salad with roasted vegetables and rice and with olive oil, lemon and herbs stirred through. Twice a week, I'll make up a big batch of salad and divide it into portions to save time.

My afternoon snack was a couple of handfuls of mixed nuts in between appointments. Clinic finished at 5pm and, after picking up my youngest daughter, I ate at around 6pm. Tonight's supper was fish with salad – I don't eat meat, so I always try to have some protein (like fish or cheese) with my evening meal.

After my daughter goes to sleep, I usually do a couple of hours' work before bed – tonight that involves writing this chapter!

I usually fast for at least ten (sometimes twelve) hours until the following morning. Time-restricted eating has been shown to be very beneficial in protecting against obesity, diabetes, cardiovascular disease and cancer.[208]

Even at the weekends, I eat similar food and at the same times. Being rigid in my routines for eating is really important in reducing migraine frequency, so I have just got used to doing this.

I cook everything from scratch and often bulk cook and freeze portions, so even when my days are really busy I know I will always have food.

It's all about striking a balance. But what does balance look like on a plate?

Think colourful, fresh ingredients, avoiding processed foods where you can. Ready meals are a lifesaver when you need something quick, but they tend to be higher in salt and other additives, plus the portion sizes can be smaller, leaving you looking for the next meal sooner than you would otherwise.

The menopause can be a period of upheaval, so try to see food as an anchor during these times. We all know we need to eat a diet packed with vitamins and minerals. But which are important during menopause? And what do we need to eat to ensure we are getting enough? Let's look at some of the key nutrients we all need to consider as the building blocks to a healthy, balanced diet.

Note: remember, this is general advice so, if you have allergies or intolerances, always follow the advice of your own specialists.

SURVEY: GOOD, GLORIOUS FOOD

Tiredness, stress and a lack of motivation to prepare nutritious meals were the key barriers to eating a balanced diet during the perimenopause and menopause, my survey found.

'I am trying to eat more healthily but often find that low mood takes me off track,' one respondent said.

Two thirds (68 per cent) said they had gained weight since the start of perimenopause or menopause but, encouragingly, a third (35 per cent) of respondents said they were trying to eat a more balanced diet.

One respondent had experienced 'gradual weight gain' but said switching to a Mediterranean style diet had helped.

'A conscious effort to reduce sugar has helped with mood and flushes,' they added.

'I now have a very low intolerance to alcohol so I either skip it altogether or end up suffering with low mood/anxiety after drinking.'

All about calcium

Calcium is a mineral that gives your bones the strength and hardness they need to cope with everyday activities.

Cast your mind back to childhood, and you may well have memories of being given milk in little cartons or glass bottles. Or if you've had children, you probably remember leaflets from healthcare professionals on the importance of calcium in building strong bones in young people.

But while it's undoubtedly crucial for growing children, our calcium needs extend far beyond childhood. With the increased risk of osteoporosis, maintaining a good calcium intake during perimenopause and menopause is so important. And while calcium is known for supporting bone health, it also serves other important functions in regulating muscle contractions, including our heartbeats and blood clotting.

How much do I need?

You should be aiming to get all the calcium you need from your diet, and adults aged nineteen to sixty-four need 700mg a day, according to UK government guidelines.[209] Not sure you are getting enough? The Royal Osteoporosis Society recommends an online calcium calculator developed by the University of Edinburgh;[210] you can use this to check whether you are getting enough calcium from what you eat and drink.

Sources of calcium

Dairy products such as milk, yoghurt, kefir (a fermented drink made from cows' milk) and cheese are all rich in calcium. But it's not all about dairy; the following foods are also calcium-rich:

- Green leafy vegetables
- Nuts and seeds
- Soft fish bones found in sardines and whitebait
- Dried fruit
- Pulses
- Tofu
- Calcium-fortified foods and drinks, such as breakfast cereals and plant-based milks (always check the label to see if they are fortified)

The lowdown on vitamin D

Vitamin D is one of those key nutrients during perimenopause and menopause – and post-menopause, too.

The primary benefit of having enough vitamin D is for the health and strength of your bones because it helps your body to absorb and use calcium, which gives them their strength and hardness.

Many researchers believe that vitamin D is vital to healthy brain function, and studies suggest it might play an important role in regulating mood and warding off anxiety and depression.[211] Vitamin D may also help to regulate insulin levels, and research has found that people with low vitamin D levels have a higher risk of developing type 2 diabetes. Vitamin D supplementation may help lower blood-sugar levels in people with type 2 diabetes and reduce the chance that prediabetes (where there are high blood-glucose levels but not enough to be classed as diabetes) develops into full-blown diabetes.[212]

Now for the science bit

Vitamin D works in a different way from other vitamins. It is more similar to a hormone and is naturally produced in the body from cholesterol when your skin is exposed to the sun. Hence, it is sometimes referred to as the 'sunshine vitamin'. It is fat-soluble (it dissolves in fats and oils) and can be stored in your body for a long time.

Note: it's important to keep in mind that all nutrients work best alongside others. Many of them depend on one another, and increased intake of one nutrient may increase your need for another. Try to make sure you have adequate amounts of calcium and magnesium to make the most of your vitamin-D supplementation.

Am I getting enough?

There are three ways to get vitamin D: through your diet, through exposure to the sun and via a supplement.

The best dietary sources of vitamin D are oily fish such as salmon, sardines, herring and mackerel, red meat, liver, egg yolks and fortified foods (such as some fat spreads and breakfast cereals). If you are vegan, there are also plant-based milks and yoghurts and some orange juices that are fortified with vitamin D. Raw chanterelle mushrooms are another source.

However, dietary sources don't generally provide adequate amounts, and a more effective way for your body to produce vitamin D is by exposing your skin to the sun. This should be at least an hour a day, when your shadow is shorter than you (so the midday sun) – which is often hard in the UK and many other countries. Because of this, UK government guidelines recommend that everyone takes 10 micrograms of a vitamin D supplement daily, throughout the year, but especially in the autumn and winter months.[213]

Vitamin D deficiency

It is estimated that about a quarter of all adults in the UK do not get enough vitamin D. People more at risk are those whose lifestyle, job or abilities mean they are predominantly indoors. Older skin makes less vitamin D, and if you are of an African-Caribbean or South Asian background, your skin takes longer to produce required amounts. If you wear clothing that covers your skin fully (say, for cultural or religious reasons), you will also be at risk of not getting enough sun exposure for vitamin D synthesis.

When vitamin D levels are very low, symptoms may include tiredness, weakness and muscle, back and bone pain. You may be more prone to infections and have poorer skin healing; your mood may be low, and you could be at risk of developing depression. If vitamin-D levels remain low for years or even decades, you may be at greater risk of type 2 diabetes, heart disease, weight gain and cancer.[214]

A word on iron

Iron is a mineral found in every cell in your body. It is an essential part of haemoglobin in red blood cells, which carries oxygen around the body. If you don't have sufficient levels of iron, your body can't make enough haemoglobin, leading to fatigue, which can affect everything from your brain function to your immune system's ability to fight off infections.

How much iron you need each day depends on your age, sex and overall health. It is not excreted from your body in urine or faeces, but is lost in blood, sweat and other secretions.

Why iron is important for women

Women need more iron than men during the years that they have periods because they lose iron in menstrual blood. After the menopause, a woman's iron needs drop as her menstrual cycle ends and recommendations of iron requirements are then the same as for men. If you are still having periods over the age of fifty, iron requirements for menstruating women still apply. If your periods stop earlier, before you are fifty (as they do for many women), your needs would be the same as for over-fifties.

The hormone oestradiol can interfere with how your body metabolises iron.[215] Many menopausal women can also have low iron even if they are not having periods. Iron levels (ferritin) can usually be measured by a blood test.

How much iron should I have every day?

The UK government recommends a daily iron intake of 14.8mg a day for women aged nineteen to fifty (or older, if still having periods) and 8.7mg a day for men and for women over fifty who are no longer having periods.[216]

Too little iron – iron-deficiency anaemia

Many people's diets do not contain adequate sources of iron; however, despite this, 95 per cent of the UK population has enough iron in their blood to not be considered iron deficient. Iron deficiency is the most common cause of anaemia world-wide. As the name suggests, it is caused by a lack of iron, often because of blood loss, and it is estimated that about 500 million people worldwide are iron deficient.[217]

Girls and women of reproductive age are particularly at risk of developing iron-deficiency anaemia, especially if they have heavy periods. It can also be a sign of unseen blood loss due to a number of conditions, such as inflammation or ulcers in the stomach or duodenum (the upper part of the small intestine). It can also be a side effect of medications such as ibuprofen or aspirin, or a common bacteria in the stomach called H pylori. It can also be caused by 'silent' bleeding from the bowel due to a polyp or even a growth, or from inflammation of the bowel (colitis). It can be a complication of coeliac disease and, on rare occasions, visible bleeding from piles can cause iron deficiency.

Often, people often don't know they are anaemic until some of the following symptoms appear:

- Feeling fatigued
- Difficulty exercising
- Shortness of breath
- Cold hands and feet
- Brittle nails or hair loss, or sores at the corner of the mouth or on the tongue

If you are concerned that you may be anaemic, you should see a healthcare professional. Diagnosing iron-deficiency anaemia usually requires a blood test and is usually treated with iron tablets and by eating iron-rich foods. Unexplained iron deficiency will require further investigation.

Left untreated, iron-deficiency anaemia can leave you at increased risk of illness and infection due to the effects on your immune system, and cardiovascular complications, such as an abnormally fast heartbeat (tachycardia) or sometimes heart failure.

Food sources of iron

Aiming to get your daily iron requirements from food is the best way to ensure your body has what it needs, as many of the foods rich in iron also contain other vitamins and minerals that will help you absorb and use it. The most easily absorbable form of iron is from meat, especially liver and kidney, and from seafood, particularly oysters, mussels and sardines. However, meat and seafood need to be eaten with vegetables rich in vitamin C to help your body absorb the iron.

Although meat and seafood are rich in iron, they should be eaten in moderation and be balanced out with plenty of other sources as well, including the following:

- Almonds, walnuts, sesame, sunflower and pumpkin seeds
- Lentils, red kidney beans, cannellini white beans, black beans, soybeans
- Dried apricots, dried figs, raisins, prunes
- Green leafy vegetables such as watercress and kale
- Jerusalem artichokes and leeks
- Parsley and thyme
- Jacket potatoes
- Eggs
- Cereals and bread with added iron (fortified)

While these foods are relatively high in iron, they are still low compared to animal-based proteins like meat and shellfish. For example, two full heads (not florets) of broccoli will give you 4.4mg of iron or 13 tablespoons of lentils (160g) will give you 5.6mg. This compares to 9mg iron for a 140g portion of lamb's liver or 3.8mg for a 140g portion of minced beef.

Foods that can adversely affect iron absorption

Some foods and drinks make it harder for your body to absorb iron, so, if you are purposefully eating iron-rich foods, you may also want to have less of the following:

- Tea
- Coffee
- Milk and dairy foods
- Foods with high levels of phytic acid, such as wholegrain cereals

Iron supplements: what you need to know

It may be beneficial to take an iron supplement, particularly if you are still having periods, or if you are not getting enough iron in your diet. You may be advised to take a supplement if you have been diagnosed with iron-deficiency anaemia, and this may be more than the recommended daily requirement. But be aware that taking more than the daily recommendation is not advised without medical supervision; high doses of iron supplements can cause nausea, vomiting and stomach pain. Iron supplements can also cause diarrhoea, dark stools or constipation; adding extra fibre to your diet or taking a stool-softener remedy can help to relieve the constipation.

Side effects of iron supplementation may be mitigated if you start with a low dose and then gradually increase it to the daily recommended amount. You can also try taking the iron supplement with food.

Should I be adding plant oestrogens to my diet?

Also known as phytoestrogens, these are plant-derived compounds that have a similar structure to human oestrogen. Phytoestrogens naturally occur in certain foods, including the following:

- Soybeans and soy-based products
- Peanuts
- Sesame seeds
- Flaxseeds
- Chickpeas
- Berries
- Barley

- Apricots
- Tea (both green and black)

You can look to up the amount of phytoestrogens in your diet, but it is worth pointing out that they do not have the same potency as the oestrogen produced by your body, so will not have a very significant effect. In addition, there is no evidence that phytoestrogens are beneficial for menopause symptoms or future health in the way that oestrogen in HRT has been shown to be. These foods are healthy for other reasons, but I would not recommend them solely to boost your oestrogen levels.

Pack in the protein

Proteins are often referred to as the building blocks of the human body. Made up of long chains of molecules known as amino acids, proteins are a key nutrient for energy, help to maintain muscle strength, make and repair cells and support wound healing. Protein also helps to keep you fuller for longer between meals by reducing levels of the hunger hormone ghrelin, while boosting levels of the appetite-regulating hormone peptide YY. We need protein throughout our lives, but during menopause it can help energy levels, which can be at a low ebb.

How much do I need?

Current guidelines are that most adults need 0.75g of protein per kilo of body weight per day: this works out for the average woman at 45g a day and 55g for men.[218] That's about two portions of meat, fish, nuts or tofu a day.

Sources of protein

- Eggs
- Milk
- Cheese
- Yoghurt
- Lean meat, such as chicken and turkey
- Fish and seafood
- Soya, such as fortified tofu and soya milks
- Beans and pulses
- Nuts and seeds

Think about fibre

A type of carbohydrate that cannot be completely broken down by human digestive enzymes, fibre passes through the body undigested. Sometimes referred to as 'roughage', fibre may not be the sexiest of foodstuffs, but it really is vital. While on its own fibre doesn't contain any calories, vitamins or minerals, it helps to keep other foods moving through the GI (gastrointestinal) tract, regulates blood sugar, keeps us feeling full and also encourages the growth of gut bacteria (more of which from Emma Ellice Flint a little later – see p. 305). Eating enough fibre will help keep you regular and fuller – which is good for those times when you feel fatigued and tempted to reach for unhealthy food choices for a quick pick-me-up.

There are two types of fibre and, as a general rule, most people need to incorporate both into their diets:

- **Soluble fibre** dissolves in water and forms a gel-like substance that slows digestion and keeps us feeling fuller for longer. It also helps to stabilise our blood-sugar levels. Soluble fibre is found in foods such as oats, barley, rye, lentils, beans, fruits and vegetables.
- **Insoluble fibre** does not dissolve in water. It adds bulk to stools and absorbs water, making them softer and easier to

pass. Sources of insoluble fibre include wholegrain foods, wholewheat flour, nuts, flaxseeds, fruits and vegetables with skins and pips intact.

How much fibre?

UK government guidelines state that adults need 30g of fibre a day.[219]

Carbohydrates and the glycaemic index (GI)

Carbohydrates can get a bad press at times. They are frequently blamed for weight gain and post-dinner slumps; and they're often the first type of food we reach for when we feel down. But not all carbs are made equal, and some are a really important energy source. They are essential at any point in your life, but especially if you are coping with fatigue during the menopause. It is generally best to obtain your carbs from vegetables, which also contain fibre and other nturients.

The glycaemic index (GI) is a rating system for carbohydrate-containing foods based on how quickly each one affects your blood-sugar level. High-GI foods can cause blood-sugar levels to rise rapidly (causing the pancreas to release more insulin) and then quickly fall. This can lead to you craving food and/or over-eating. The following are high-GI:

- Sugar and sugary foods
- Sugary soft drinks
- White bread
- Potatoes
- White rice

Low-GI foods, in comparison, are broken down more slowly and cause smaller rises in your blood sugar. They will keep you satisfied for longer and encourage your body to burn fat.

Examples include the following:

- Some fruit and vegetables (including apples, pears, blueberries, strawberries, asparagus, mushrooms, spinach and onions)
- Pulses
- Wholegrain foods, such as porridge oats

Choose your fats wisely

When I talk to women about their diets, I always ask about how much fat they are eating. A common answer is, 'Oh, too much', so then I rephrase the question to ask how much *good* fat they include in their diets.

Like carbs, fats have a bad reputation. Yet they are vital for energy and to absorb vitamins – like vitamin D (needed for healthy bones, which is so important heading into the menopause and beyond). They are also a source of essential fatty acids (known as omega 3 and omega 6) that help to keep your brain healthy.

However, some fats are better than others – and it's important to know the difference for a balanced diet. Eating too much of the unhealthier fats can lead to weight gain – which can be an issue during the menopause, as we cover a little later on in this chapter – and raise your risk of developing cardiovascular disease.

So which fats are ok to eat on a regular basis, and which are better eaten in moderation?

Let's look at the four main types:

- **Saturated fats** are usually solid at room temperature and are mainly found in animal products like butter, cheese, fatty cuts of meat and in processed foods like sausages, hamburgers and cakes. Eating too much saturated fat can raise the level of LDL or 'bad' cholesterol in your blood and increase the risk of cardiovascular disease.

- **Trans fats** are found in small amounts in some foods and, like saturated fats, can raise LDL cholesterol levels in the blood. They are found in processed foods like cakes, biscuits and takeaway foods. These should, ideally, be avoided.

Tip: check your food labels, as trans fats can also be listed as 'hydrogenated vegetable fats/oil'.

- **Monounsaturated fats** are healthy fats that help to protect your heart by maintaining levels of HDL, or 'good' cholesterol, and reducing LDL cholesterol in your blood. They are found in olive oil, avocados and nuts, including Brazil nuts, almonds and peanuts.
- **Polyunsaturated fats** are another type of unsaturated fat that includes omega 3, found in fatty fish like salmon and mackerel, and in smaller amounts in plant oils like rapeseed, soya, flax and linseed, walnuts and omega 3-enriched eggs. Plant oils are also a source of omega 6.

How much fat do I really need?

Government guidelines say women should eat no more than 70g of fat a day, to include no more than 20g of saturated fat and no more than 5g of trans fat.[220] So you can go ahead and eat fat, but it's about making some informed choices.

When I was writing this chapter, I undertook a bit of a cupboard audit, looking up the nutritional values of some of my family's favourite foods. One of the things I checked was avocados. I love them in salads, either chopped up or blended to make a creamy dressing; my family loves them mashed up with a pinch of black pepper and chilli flakes and used as a toast topping. When you look up the fat content of a medium avocado, it contains 22g of fat – almost a third of the recommended daily intake.[221] This might set alarm bells ringing, but if you look at the nutritional breakdown, the 22g is made up of 15g monounsaturated, 4g polyunsaturated and only 3g saturated fat, making it a good choice for getting those healthy fats into your diet.

Now, let's compare that avocado to a cheeseburger. A cheeseburger contains 12g of fat – just over half of the fat in an avocado. But looking more closely at the nutritional breakdown, it contains 5.5g of saturated fat – nearly double the amount of an avocado.

The bottom line? Fats are essential – but look to unsaturated fats in the main to get your daily allowance.

CASE STUDY: I CAME BACK FROM ROCK BOTTOM . . . AND WON PROMOTION – MARIA'S STORY

Maria has had a long and distinguished career in policing, but during the COVID-19 pandemic she was depressed and clinically obese. Here, she shares how she lost weight and turned her life around.

'In 2018, when I was forty-eight, I started experiencing low moods. I knew it was depression, so I went to see my GP, but they wouldn't prescribe me HRT for the menopause, due to my history of having had a blood clot when I was thirty-seven. Instead, they told me to look for natural ways to cope with my symptoms or be prepared to take antidepressants.

'Things went from bad to worse. I've always been very sporty since childhood, but at the same time struggled with my weight. I've tried every diet and eating plan you can think of, but nothing worked. I'd lose a bit of weight initially, but then I'd put it back on – and more.

'Around the start of the COVID-19 pandemic, I weighed 93kg. I was obese, stressed out and anxious.

'Policing is a high-pressure job, and I had a lot of responsibility – but I'd always managed. Now, it felt like it was increasingly hard to cope. I remember one meeting where I burst into tears, which was completely out of character for me.

'I should've taken some time out then, but I wouldn't allow myself. I was worried about what others would think if I did. When I was off shift, I turned to food and alcohol for comfort. Anything carby was usually my go-to, and I was definitely drinking too much, averaging a bottle of wine every night.

'I tried to make changes, cutting out alcohol completely and focusing on exercise. But in July 2020, following a 26-mile bike ride, I developed a blood clot in my leg. I was diagnosed with deep-vein thrombosis (DVT) and given blood-thinning medication to deal with the clot.

'Even then, I carried on working. The following month, I was working from home and in a virtual meeting when I started to feel unwell. I looked down at my wristwatch, which measures my heart rate. My resting heart rate was 200 beats per minute (usually, it's 50).

'I left the meeting and headed to the emergency department. I was panicking that my recent blood clot had travelled to my heart or lungs. Doctors diagnosed me with supraventricular tachycardia (SVT), a condition when your heart suddenly beats faster than normal. Whilst waiting for further tests I continued to work, but my anxiety increased.

'A few weeks later, I broke down in tears to a close friend. The reality hit me. I was at rock bottom.

'My doctor signed me off from work. There was no way I would have been able to work, as the slightest thing would reduce me to tears. I even looked into taking early retirement because I was convinced my career was over.

'I knew I had to do something about my weight and that calorie counting or fad diets were no longer an option. I'm a keen cyclist and saw Olympic cyclist Chris Froome on Facebook using a health gadget called Lumen to measure his metabolism.

'With the time to recover and focus on my health, I gave it a try, and used the nutritional plan on the accompanying app. The weight started to fall off. By September 2021, I had lost four stone. At the same time, I started to take HRT.

'My energy was back, I was sleeping better and my weight was in the healthy range for body mass index. I felt more confident than I had in years.

'Last year, I went on holiday to Mallorca and packed six bikinis – I'd never worn a bikini before in my life.

'Career-wise, I returned to work in April 2021 and when an opportunity came up to apply for a temporary senior post for the Police, I applied. I wouldn't have dreamed of doing that even a year before. The interview went well, and I remember thinking to myself afterwards that even if I didn't get it, I was proud of how far I had come in such a short space of time. When I found out I had got the job, it was an incredible feeling.

'I've gone from someone who was obese, with SVT, suffering from acute perimenopausal stress and burned out at work to winning a temporary promotion. And I'm determined to help others. I have just set up a steering group at work to embed managing and supporting employees going through menopause in the workplace. I've also been appointed National Police Chief's Council lead for menopause for UK policing.'

Let's talk about weight gain

Weight gain during the perimenopause and menopause is one of those physical symptoms that can have a real knock-on effect on self-esteem, body confidence and motivation.

It can be so disheartening to feel bloated and uncomfortable when you put on unwanted weight. Feeling sluggish or the realisation that a favourite outfit you wanted to wear for a special event no longer fits can be pretty miserable.

Often, women will say while their eating habits haven't changed, the weight has crept up on them, particularly around the waist. For others, physical symptoms like joint pains and vaginal dryness mean they don't exercise as much as they did previously for fear of exacerbating their symptoms.

Extensive evidence shows that changes in body composition, including the loss of lean body mass, accumulation of fat mass and redistribution of the fat (adipose) tissue in the abdominal area, occur for many women during the menopause.[222] These and other metabolic changes that occur at this time lead to a greater risk of insulin resistance (increasing glucose levels and increased risk of type 2 diabetes) and also a rise in cholesterol.[223,224]

When we've had a bad day at work or cross words with a loved one, or we're simply feeling a bit low, we often will turn to food as a treat. And invariably, something sugary, salty or fatty will hit the spot. Of course, an occasional treat is fine, but this habit can become ingrained, and we find ourselves using food as a crutch without even thinking.

Why have I put on weight?

While we often point the finger at our own behaviours, there is much more to menopausal weight gain than you might think.

Hormones and weight gain

During the perimenopause and menopause, our bodies look to combat decreasing levels of oestrogen by trying to obtain it elsewhere – chiefly a different form of the hormone produced by fat cells. This type of oestrogen, oestrone, is less effective than oestradiol and also more inflammatory in your body. Oestrone is not associated with benefits in the body, as it works very differently to oestradiol.

Many women find that they start to develop a 'spare tyre' in response to this and might also have strong cravings for foods high in sugar or unhealthy fats, which the body will, in turn, lay down as oestrone-producing abdominal fat.

There may also be changes to your visceral (internal) fat. There is evidence that the accumulation of visceral rather than subcutaneous (under the skin) fat is associated with a greater cardiometabolic risk – meaning an increased risk of heart disease and type 2 diabetes.[225] Your sympathetic nervous system is the part of the nervous system that increases heart rate, blood pressure and breathing rate. It also causes blood vessels to narrow and reduces digestive juices. The sympathetic nervous system is supported by oestrogen, so low levels can trigger a fight/flight/

freeze reaction (your body's way of facing a perceived threat). This stress reaction also releases the stress hormones adrenaline and cortisol.

Adrenaline can cause symptoms such as an increase in heart and breathing rates, dry mouth and butterflies in your stomach, while cortisol causes your body to release glucose for a burst of energy to allow the body to 'flee'. When this glucose is not used for physical activity, it triggers the release of insulin, which can then package the glucose away as fat.

Less exercise due to joint pains

Lower levels of oestrogen and testosterone can often cause wide-spread muscle and joint pains, and many women will reduce their day-to-day exercise because of this.

Poor sleep . . . and hunger hormones

Oestrogen deficiency can disturb sleep patterns for a number of reasons: hot flushes and night sweats, as well as disruption to the sleep hormone melatonin and raised cortisol levels. Declining oestrogen and also testosterone levels are also likely to be contributing factors to sleep disruption during the perimeno-pause and menopause.[226]

Anxiety can manifest at night as well, due to the cortisol imbalance, and many women can wake during the night with hunger cravings when they never did before.

Leptin and ghrelin are two other hormones that are closely linked to weight. Leptin acts as an appetite suppressant and ghrelin is an appetite stimulant. Increased fat in the body can cause leptin resistance, which means that the normal signals to let you know you are full become disrupted.

Sleep also has an important part to play in the regulation of these two hormones; poor sleep can increase ghrelin, making you feel hungry, and decrease leptin, which stops you from feeling full.

Low testosterone

Declining testosterone levels can lead to a decrease in muscle mass and lower energy levels. This, in turn, can reduce your baseline metabolic rate; fewer calories are burned, even with the same nutritional intake as before your perimenopause.

Neurotransmitters – such as dopamine, oxytocin and serotonin – are chemicals that often impact on mood and the reward centres in your brain. We know that fluctuating oestrogen and testosterone can influence the levels of these neurotransmitters.[227] Dopamine is often released when thinking about a 'reward' or pleasurable experience and can be linked to repeated patterns of behaviour, such as comfort eating at the end of a stressful day. Serotonin is responsible for improving your mood and can be affected by fluctuating hormones. It has an effect on appetite regulation and, as well as being produced in your brain, it is also produced in your gut.

Changes to your metabolism

In a study I was involved in, led by epidemiologist and science writer Professor Tim Spector and his team, we demonstrated that menopausal women are more likely to weigh more, eat more sugary foods, have higher levels of glucose and insulin and to report sleep difficulties. Menopausal women were also more likely to have higher levels of postprandial glycaemia (raised glucose levels after eating). We also found that those women taking HRT had less visceral fat, lower glucose and insulin levels and differences in their gut microbiomes. We are doing more research into this important area.[228]

EXPERT VIEW
Set yourself some SMART goals –
Dr Sally Norton, medical doctor,
Weight-loss consultant and the UK's first
female weight-loss surgeon

As a medical doctor and weight-loss consultant, Dr Sally has helped thousands of patients who have struggled with their weight. As one of the 'balance+ gurus' on my app, she is passionate about helping women to maintain a healthy weight, while navigating the additional challenges of perimenopause and menopause.

When the waistband is tightening, it is tempting to set yourself a weight-loss goal with the help of the latest diet in a newspaper supplement, or to give the diet that has worked for your best friend a go.

The trouble with a goal like this is that it is simply too rigid. You set yourself up for failure when your willpower runs out. Instead, it's time to think smart using SMART goal setting.

S: specific

Intentions need to be specific and, in my opinion, small, so you can achieve them and build upon them. Most people trying to lose weight will rely on the scales to set their goal, but that often leads to rapid loss of motivation. In fact, my weight-loss programme doesn't focus on the scales at all, but uses specific healthier-eating goals, or even sleep and relaxation, which can help weight loss by restoring hormonal balance.

M: measurable

Can you measure your goals easily? We all need things to aim for, whether it is an essay deadline at school, or a savings goal towards a big purchase. This motivates us and keeps us on track – and it's also useful when it comes to weight loss.

A: attainable

There's no point in having a goal that you are never going to achieve, so ensure that you are being realistic in your goal setting. If you know you have a tiring week at work, cut yourself some slack and set yourself some less taxing but useful intentions.

R: relevant

Any goals you set to keep you on track towards your ultimate goal need to be relevant. You might want to focus on better nutrition, more sleep, drinking less alcohol or lowering stress to help you achieve sustainable, easier weight loss.

T: time-limited

You need to set a time limit for achieving these goals, or they can drift. Ensure you have a clear, attainable deadline.

That's SMART goals sorted. But if you really want to succeed, make them SMARTER:

E: enjoyable

When your goals are enjoyable, they are easier to achieve. Can you enlist a friend to help you on your weight-loss journey? Or if you have children, involving them by trying out new recipes in the kitchen could be a fun activity.

R: rewarding

Losing weight in a sustainable, fad-free way has rewards in itself, such as reducing your risk of diabetes, heart disease, some cancers and more. In addition, it will almost certainly improve your mental health. Think creatively about how to reward yourself when you reach your goals (obviously not something that will undo all your good work). It could be coffee with a friend, a trip to the cinema, or buying a new book or something else you have had your eye on for a while.

Trust your gut: the role of gut health in menopause

Your gastrointestinal tract is a series of organs that form part of your digestive system, including our oesophagus, stomach and intestines. It helps to digest, absorb and process all the nutrients and water from what you eat and drink.

Within your gut are trillions of living organisms, collectively known as the gut microbiome. Teeming with these bacteria, viruses and fungi, the gut microbiome can affect your hormones, metabolism and immunity, and what you eat can directly influence the delicate balance, as Emma Ellice Flint describes below.

Your gut microbiome is incredibly important, and the last two decades have seen a great surge of interest in this fascinating area.

EXPERT VIEW
Five reasons to boost your gut health – Emma Ellice Flint,
Clinical nutritionist, chef and author

As a nutritionist, I believe the foundation of all health, balance and wellbeing is a healthy gut. Here are five reasons why we need to nurture it, and some suggestions for how to incorporate more gut-friendly foods into your diet.

Finally, I'll be sharing a selection of delicious, nourishing recipes to help you put these principles into practice.

1. Boost your mood

The food choices we make each day can affect our gut microbiome either positively or negatively. The beneficial microbiota (the collection of micro-organisms living in the microbiome in the gastrointestinal tract) thrives when we eat foods that encourage its health, while incorrect foods may not only foster a hostile environment for it, but also encourage unwanted bacteria to thrive instead. The gut microbiota communicates with the brain, and vice versa, via several neural pathways. Amazingly, some gut microbiota can produce their own neurotransmitters – hormones that can communicate directly with the brain in its own language.

Through this connection our moods can influence, and be influenced by, the gut's condition – happiness, positivity, excitement and optimism are affected by a healthy microbiota, while tendencies to grumpiness, anger, anxiety and tearfulness may reflect an out-of-balance gut microbiome.

2. Combat stress

The wall of the small intestine is covered with villi – small, finger-like projections that increase its surface area and capacity to absorb nutrients from food. Studies have shown that chronic stress can reduce the length of the villi, so at these times it's important to boost our 'good' gut microbiota. These produce small fatty acids such as butyrate, which feed the villi and encourage them to grow larger and more robust, so increasing their absorption of nutrients, vitamins, minerals and phytochemicals, and also making them less likely to take in unwanted substances. That's a win for the body, as it has access to more of the beneficial stuff from our food. By boosting your gut health, these villi can remain strong and nourished to do their job, even when you're stressed.

3. Boost your immune system

Both our friendly microbiota and the gut lining are instrumental in helping to prevent us getting sick, or in reducing the severity of an illness and complications, such as secondary infections. But here's the tricky part: for those of us following the norms of Western or European culture, our guts tend to have a lower bacterial diversity. In part, this is due to a more widespread use of antibiotics, which kill both the good and the bad bacteria in the gut. Also at fault is a typically low-fibre diet, containing very few prebiotic foods (these encourage the growth of beneficial bacteria in the gut), which deprives any remaining beneficial bacteria of the nutrition they need to thrive and multiply again after periods of antibiotic treatment. To help break a potentially vicious cycle of ill health, it's important to increase the level of prebiotic and probiotic fermented foods in our daily diets. The resulting vigour of our guts will help make our immune systems more resilient.

4. Prevent weight gain

People who are overweight or obese tend to have a different gut microbiota profile to those in a healthier weight range, which has led scientists to theorise that improving the microbiota could benefit weight loss. Trials were conducted on mice, transferring gut bacteria from thin mice into overweight mice, with the result that the overweight mice lost weight.[229] Extrapolating that example to the human body, it's possible to conclude that the health of the microbiota of an overweight person affects their gut's ability to process food efficiently, so the body is no longer the fat-burning machine nature designed. Prebiotic foods promote good gut bacteria – and these same foods also happen to help us feel fuller and satisfied.

5. Energy boost

Unhealthy eating patterns and an out-of-balance gut microbiome can lead to subclinical infection, causing mild inflammation without you even knowing it. Sufferers of such inflammation may experience seemingly unrelated symptoms, like fatigue, hormonal imbalance, weight gain, lack of energy and being 'fuzzy headed'. Research indicates that chronic-fatigue sufferers often present with a differing or reduced microbiome profile when compared to those without the condition.[230] Related studies have shown a measurable improvement in fatigue symptoms when specific probiotics are administered. Even without a diagnosed explanation for fatigue, patients in my clinic who have added prebiotic and probiotic foods to their diets report that they have increased energy.

So which foods boost gut health?

This question is a tricky one, since there are particular foods that are great for our gut microbiota but they can trigger gastrointestinal disturbances in some people. In my clinic, I work with people to discover which foods would be good for their guts and overall feelings of wellbeing and vitality, but also well tolerated by them.

- Prebiotic foods include: garlic, onions, asparagus, chicory, radicchio, artichoke, cocoa, ginger, cabbage, fennel, beet-root, bananas, blueberries, apples, nuts, herbs, seeds and spices.
- Probiotic foods include: kefir, live yoghurt, kombucha, sauerkraut, kimchi, natto and live apple cider vinegar.

Then there are foods that particularly help boost the layer lining the gut wall where these microbes live, and others again that help with 'cleansing' it – an important step often overlooked by people wanting to improve their gut health, and one that helps to reduce inflammation. These foods include bone broth, flax/linseeds and oats.

We've been through the theory and now for the fun part – trying some delicious new recipes. On the following pages are suggestions for tasty, filling breakfasts, lunches and suppers. Enjoy!

BREAKFAST

Mood-boosting berry smoothie

....

If you are someone who likes a breakfast smoothie, this is for you.

Serves 1

225g fresh or frozen berries of your choice, such as blackberries, blue-
    berries, raspberries or strawberries (use frozen berries if you prefer a
    thicker smoothie)

225g natural unsweetened kefir, yoghurt or plant-based yoghurt

1 heaped tbsp flaxseeds or linseeds

1 heaped tbsp oats

1 tsp natural vanilla extract, or vanilla seeds scraped from ¼ of a pod

1 pitted date or 2tsp honey, 100 per cent pure maple syrup or brown rice
    syrup, if you want to add sweetness

Method

Put all ingredients in a blender and mix until smooth and thick. For
a thinner consistency, add some water to loosen the mixture.

Pink oats with kefir

....

(Vegetarian)

Fast and pretty, these oats are a smart breakfast choice for so
many reasons. The berries contain phytonutrients that act like anti-
oxidants in the body; there's prebiotic, gut-friendly fibre from the
oats and ground flaxseeds, prebiotics from the kefir/yoghurt and
anti-inflammatory oils from the nuts and seeds. Plus, calcium is

found in most of the ingredients, particularly the dairy – so beneficial for bone health during the perimenopause and menopause.

Serves 1

115g fresh or frozen and defrosted mixed dark berries (I like a mixture of
   blackberries and blueberries)

15g ground flaxseeds or linseeds

27g whole rolled oats

2 heaped tbsp kefir, natural unsweetened yoghurt or a calcium-fortified
   plant-based yoghurt

1 tsp grated fresh ginger or ¼ tsp ground cinnamon

20g raw almonds

Method

1. In a bowl, mash up the berries with the kefir/yoghurt and
    ground flax- or linseeds. If the mixture becomes a bit thick, add
    some water or extra yoghurt.
2. Add the ginger or cinnamon.
3. Sprinkle over the almonds.
4. Eat straight away or, if making the night before, stir in about 4
    tablespoons of water and store in an airtight container in the
    fridge overnight. Soaking the oats can make them easier to
    digest if you can't tolerate raw oats.

LUNCH

Roasted beetroot and cauliflower salad with a creamy tahini dressing

....

(Vegetarian, gluten-free, wheat-free and low GI)

This salad is a great lunch or even dinner option, as it is so tasty, nutritious and filling, and beetroot and cauliflower both support gut function. If you want to add some protein to this dish, try fish, firm tofu or eggs.

Serves 2

For the salad:

320g raw beetroot

2 tbsp extra virgin olive oil

½ large cauliflower (about 600g) washed and cut into small florets

30g almonds

1 tbsp cumin seeds

2 tbsp pumpkin seeds

Handful of parsley leaves

Salt and freshly ground pepper

For the dressing:

1 tbsp lemon juice

1 heaped tbsp tahini

1 heaped tbsp unsweetened natural yoghurt

Method

1. Preheat the oven to 200°C/180°C fan.
2. Chop the stems off the beetroot and thoroughly wash off any soil – no need to peel them. Then cut into wedges and toss with 1 tablespoon of the oil, salt and pepper.
3. Put the beetroot wedges on a baking tray and roast in the oven for 30–40 minutes or until slightly soft to the touch. Tip: always aim to under- rather than overcook beetroot to help retain the nutrients.
4. Toss the cauliflower in the remaining olive oil with a good pinch of salt and pepper. Put on a separate baking tray and roast in the oven for 25 minutes, or until the cauliflower is slightly golden around the edges.
5. For the last 5 minutes of cooking time, add the almonds, cumin and pumpkin seeds to the trays to lightly roast.
6. Remove both trays from the oven and allow the beetroot, cauliflower, almonds and seeds to cool to room temperature.
7. In a large salad bowl, mix the dressing ingredients together. If the mixture looks too thick, add a little water. The aim is to get to the consistency of thin custard.
8. Chop the parsley and add to the salad bowl.
9. Add the beetroot, cauliflower, almonds, cumin and pumpkin seed mix to the salad bowl. Using your hands, gently mix the dressing through the vegetables before serving.

Mint, avocado and bean salad with crispy fish

This refreshing, nutrient-dense salad contains plenty of healthy fats to help brain function.

Serves 2

For the crispy fish:

1 large fish fillet, approximately 240g (I like to use a chunkier fish, such as monkfish or salmon)

20g coarse polenta meal or cornmeal

Pinch of salt

1 tbsp dried oregano

Pinch of black pepper and/or chilli flakes

1 tbsp extra virgin olive oil

For the salad:

200g cucumber, skin on

Large handful of mint leaves

Large handful of fresh dill

75g brown rice, quinoa or lentils, cooked and cooled

75g fresh or frozen edamame beans, podded (you can substitute with fresh or frozen broad beans, fava beans or peas)

1 avocado, peeled and cut into chunks

1 tbsp lemon juice

2 tbsp extra virgin olive oil

40g pumpkin seeds

Method

....

1. Using a sharp knife, carefully slice through the fish fillet, so you end up with smaller, thinner chunks or slices.

2. Mix the polenta or cornmeal with the oregano and salt and pepper (and/or chilli flakes). Coat the fish pieces with the polenta mixture.

3. Heat a large frying pan or skillet on medium–low and add the oil.

4. Place the coated fish in the pan and cook for about 2 minutes. Turn and cook for a further 2 minutes, or until cooked through to your liking. Remove from the heat.

5. Using a mandolin or large potato peeler, cut the cucumber into really thin strips and place in a large bowl.

6. Finely chop the mint leaves and dill and add to the cucumber, then add the rice, quinoa or lentils and the edamame beans to the bowl.

7. Mix together the lemon juice and olive oil with the avocado and add to the bowl, gently mixing everything together.

8. Stack the salad on to your serving plates, scatter over the pumpkin seeds and flake the fish on top.

DINNER

Sesame-crusted salmon with ginger and mint slaw

....

(Low GI)

This dish contains plenty of vitamin C and protein, which help to nourish the skin, plus the anti-inflammatory oils in the salmon and seeds also help to protect the skin's integrity during perimeno-pause and menopause, when it can become drier and thinner.

Serves 2

250g salmon fillet, cut into chunks or small strips (you can substitute salmon for firm tofu cut into chunks)

2 tbsp sesame seeds

1 tsp extra virgin olive oil

4 spring onions, roughly chopped

For the slaw:

200g broccoli, cut into very small florets

Large handful of fresh mint, chopped

120g red or white cabbage, or wombok/napa cabbage, very thinly sliced

1 tbsp thinly sliced pickled ginger

A handful of cooked lentils, quinoa or brown rice (optional)

For the dressing:

1 tbsp freshly grated ginger

1 heaped tsp miso paste or powder

1 tbsp live apple cider vinegar

1 tbsp soy sauce or tamari soy sauce (which is wheat-free) or a large pinch of salt

1 tbsp extra virgin olive oil

Method

1. Mix all the dressing ingredients together, using a fork to smash the miso paste into the mixture. Set aside.
2. Toss the salmon with the sesame seeds to roughly coat all over.

THE DEFINITIVE GUIDE TO THE PERIMENOPAUSE AND MENOPAUSE

3. Blanch the broccoli in boiling water for about 2 minutes, or steam for about 4 minutes. Refresh in cold water to prevent the broccoli from cooking longer, then drain.

4. Mix all the slaw ingredients together in a bowl, but don't add the dressing until just before serving, as the cabbage will wilt.

5. Set a large frying pan or skillet on a high heat and add the oil and spring onions. Cook for about 30 seconds to just scorch the outside of the onions, not to cook them. Remove from the pan and add to the slaw.

6. Add the salmon to the pan and sear on each side for about 30 seconds. Remove from the pan and turn off the heat. (How long you cook the salmon for depends on whether you prefer it to be cooked all the way through or left slightly undercooked in the centre – cut one of the chunks open to check if unsure.) If substituting salmon with firm tofu, simply toss the tofu with the sesame seeds; it is already cooked, so only needs warming through in the pan.

7. When ready to serve, toss the slaw with the dressing and divide between two plates, then top with the seared salmon.

Comfort in a bowl

....

(Vegetarian, gluten-free, low GI)

Made in minutes, but designed to be eaten slowly, this nourishing, warming bowl is my idea of comfort food. I first made this recipe during the COVID-19 lockdown and it's become a firm favourite – not only for its taste and texture, but also because I know it is great for my gut health. It's worth noting that if you are suffering from poor sleep during menopause, this recipe can also help with this

NUTRITION DURING THE PERIMENOPAUSE AND MENOPAUSE

because it contains complex, slow-release carbohydrates and protein, both of which help to gently balance blood-glucose levels.

Serves 2

2 tbsp extra virgin olive oil, plus a little extra

1 tsp cumin seeds

1 large purple onion (approximately 130g), peeled and chopped

½ large broccoli head (approximately 150g), finely chopped

¼ long red chilli (these tend to be milder), finely chopped

1 garlic glove, crushed

1 tsp ginger, coarsely grated

100g chopped leafy greens, such as kale or chard

100g chopped white cabbage

15g raw almonds, roughly chopped

15g pumpkin seeds

200g cooked brown rice or quinoa

120g cooked chickpeas

2 large eggs (or some firm tofu, if you want to increase protein)

Salt and pepper

Sauerkraut or kimchi (optional)

Method

....

1. Pop the oil, cumin seeds and onion in a large frying pan. Cook gently on a medium heat, until the onion begins to soften.

2. Add the broccoli, chilli, garlic and ginger. Gently cook for a couple of minutes, stirring occasionally

3. Add the greens, cabbage, almonds and pumpkin seeds and toss to combine. Allow the greens to wilt, then stir in the cooked rice/quinoa and chickpeas to warm.

4.   Season with salt and pepper and then tip out into two bowls.

5.   Using the same frying pan, add a little drizzle of olive oil and fry the two large eggs, until crispy on the edges, then top the bowls with an egg on each. Alternatively, crumble through some cooked firm tofu for added protein.

6.   Top with some live sauerkraut or kimchi, if desired, for added gut benefits.

SNACKS

Calcium-rich Parmesan oatcakes

....

(Vegetarian, wheat-free)

Perfect as a snack or to accompany a nourishing salad, these nutritious oatcakes are a great source of calcium to support bone health during perimenopause and menopause, plus they contain soluble and insoluble fibre, which help to keep your gut happy.

Makes 15–20 oatcakes

120g whole rolled oats

100g seeds (try pumpkin, sesame and sunflower)

20g flaxseeds or linseeds (these can be ground)

Large pinch of sea salt flakes, plus ½ tsp for decorating

5 tbsp extra virgin olive oil

Large pinch of cayenne pepper or cumin seeds (optional)

25g freshly grated vegetarian hard cheese (or if not vegetarian, you could use Parmesan instead)

5–6 tbsp water

Method

1. Preheat the oven to 200°C/180°C fan.
2. Put the oats and all the seeds into a food processor and blitz, until they form a crumb (but not as fine as flour).
3. Add the large pinch of sea salt flakes, olive oil, cayenne or cumin (if using), Parmesan and water and blend until a dough-like ball is formed.
4. Place a large piece of baking parchment on a work surface and tip the dough out on to the paper.
5. Place another piece of paper on top of the dough. Using a rolling pin or similar, roll out the dough until it is about 5mm thick for thin, crisp oatcakes or 1.5cm for softer, thicker ones.
6. Use a cookie cutter to cut out the oatcakes or cut similar-sized squares, using a sharp knife.
7. Line a large baking sheet with baking parchment and place the oatcakes on top – they can be placed close together since they will not spread while baking. Bake for 15 minutes for thin oatcakes, and 20 minutes for thicker ones.
8. Remove from the oven and leave to cool completely before moving and scattering with the rest of the sea salt flakes.

Artichoke and chickpea dip

(Vegetarian)

This Mediterranean-style dip not only tastes delicious, but has lots of ingredients to see you through the menopause transition: fibre for gut health, anti-inflammatory oil and prebiotic vegetables to support your gut microbiome. Eat it with cut raw vegetables, add a dollop to a salad or use as a spread on oatcakes or wholegrain bread.

Serves 4

250g chickpeas

3 tbsp extra virgin olive oil

1 leek, about 150g once trimmed

1 garlic clove, peeled and crushed

3cm knob of ginger, grated

Handful of parsley leaves, washed

180g cooked artichoke hearts from a jar or tin

Good pinch of salt and pepper

Method

1. Cook your chickpeas according to the packet instructions.
2. Trim the green part off the leek and discard, chop the remaining white part, rinse to remove any dirt or grit and drain well.
3. Put the oil in a large saucepan over a low heat.
4. Add the leek, pop a lid on the pan and cook slowly for approximately 5 minutes, until the leek is soft, then tip into a food processor.
5. Add the garlic, ginger, chickpeas, parsley, artichoke hearts, salt and pepper to the food processor and blend really well, until creamy. Add some more olive oil, chickpea liquid or water, if needed, to achieve the creamy consistency.

EXPERT VIEW

Eating your way to better health – Dr Rupy Aujla,
NHS Doctor and Founder of the Doctor's Kitchen

Before moving on to our next chapter, which is all about work, I wanted to leave the final word to Dr Rupy Aujla.

I spent a really enjoyable afternoon in 2022 talking to Rupy for his Doctor's Kitchen podcast. His personal story is genuinely inspiring, and I went away from our chat feeling so energised: he truly believes in the power of good food, as do I.

About ten years ago I fell ill. I was suffering from atrial fibrillation (an irregular and often abnormally fast heartbeat), and, after many tests, I was told to have an ablation procedure.

It was this that sparked a change in my lifestyle. The power of food and healthy living isn't taught in medical school, and it took my own experience to realise just how much of an impact nutrition can have. The driving force behind The Doctor's Kitchen was the idea of creating motivating, exciting and accessible recipes that encourage people to recognise food as an important health intervention. Now I'm trying to understand how we can equip the modern doctor to feel confident having conversations about food in a clinical environment.

Hundreds of studies in nutritional-science literature across multiple organisations around the world all point to the same assumption: the more fruits, vegetables, nuts and seeds in your diet, the lower the risk of disease across many areas, including cancer, heart disease, diabetes, eye disease, mental health and more.

Food and menopause

So how can what you eat enable you to have a better perimeno-pause or menopause?

Focusing your meals on plants and eating a greater variety of them is the mantra I've been reciting through all my books and recipes, and the same is true for the menopause.

When we examine the research looking at fruit and vegetables and health outcomes, the trend is fairly clear. There is a 'dose response' to eating vegetables, which, simply put, means the more the better. With each incremental increase in consumption, greater health protection is achieved. Everything from a simple carrot to your basic apple is brimming with chemicals like quercetin and carotene, known to benefit health.

And it's these simple, affordable and accessible ingredients that are key to good health. Eating plates of a variety of colour-ful plants is the easiest way to guarantee a complete range of micronutrients from food in its whole form.

The most important message I want you to take away is that it's not about focusing solely on individual ingredients and their properties. It's your dietary pattern over time, and making sure you eat whole foods to benefit from the incredible orchestra of molecules we find in food.

Let's take spinach, for example: yes, most of us will know it contains iron, but spinach also has vitamin K, folate, nitrates, polyphenols and a collection of plant chemicals with antioxi-dants. So if we can achieve more plants, fibre, colours, variety, minimally processed foods and a way of sticking to this way of eating long-term, then we can benefit immune, brain, skin, heart health and more, as demonstrated by thousands of research studies looking at these associations.

12

Menopause and Work

Four things you will learn in this chapter:

1. How menopause can impact your working life

2. Your workplace rights, and key questions to ask to secure the support you need

3. How to talk to your boss about your menopause

4. How you can help your staff, if you're a line manager

It was the end of another long, busy day seeing patients at the GP surgery where I worked. The final appointment had just finished, and the surgery doors were closed. In my consulting room, I put my head in my hands and let out a long sigh. But it wasn't a sigh of relief. It was one of frustration. Frustration because I knew my day's work was far from over. While medical appointments are all too brief, lasting just minutes, I had paperwork to catch up on, patient referrals to look over, emails to respond to . . . the list felt endless.

The paperwork had always been there, but earlier in my career it felt doable. But as a brain-fogged perimenopausal woman, that admin felt like a mountain I no longer had the energy to climb.

I truly loved my work as a GP. I enjoyed the variety of patients and the chance to make a positive difference to the health of a whole community. People see their GP as a person they can confide in – someone they can turn to when they need help and advice – and as a healthcare professional, it has never been lost on me what a huge privilege it is to be part of people's lives in that way. It's the same feeling I have about the patients I help every day with their menopause.

Helping people was exactly why I was drawn to medicine in the first place. But my working days as a perimenopausal GP were plagued by a knot of anxiety in my stomach that my brain fog and fatigue would catch me out. Was that prescription right? Had I given the correct advice to my last patient? Had I taken in what my colleague had just said to me? There were times before HRT when I felt overwhelmed with it all.

I had worked hard through medical school, and harder still when my daughters were born to keep going with my career. But here I was at a real crossroads. Could I cope with juggling home, work and looking after my health? I really wasn't sure, and that self-doubt made me feel like a failure.

Yet my experience is far from unusual. On a daily basis, in my clinic and on social media, I hear stories time and time again of aspirations and ambitions dashed and menopausal women being sidelined in the workplace.

My survey on menopause and the workplace (the findings of which I will be sharing later in this chapter – see p. 326) shows how crippling menopause symptoms and a lack of support are ruining women's work lives, forcing them to take time off or even quit their jobs altogether. Why is this?

It's because employers are failing to get a grip on the seismic impact the menopause can have, even though it makes good business sense to do so. At mid-life, women should be at the pinnacle of their careers, but instead they are disappearing from the workforce. An estimated 14 million working days a year in the UK alone are lost to menopause symptoms.[231]

So yes – it is vital that employers recognise menopause and put policies in place to support their workforce. But employer support is only part of the story. Just as important is women taking control of their own menopause, advocating for themselves and receiving individualised care, rather than simply living with potentially career-ruining symptoms, such as memory problems, low mood, fatigue and anxiety.

For far too long menopausal women have been faced with an impossible choice: struggle on with often debilitating symptoms or leave behind the careers they have worked so hard for. So this chapter is about redressing that dilemma, giving you the tools and information to stay in your job, plus there is advice for employers on how to make their organisations places where menopausal women can thrive and remain on the career ladder.

SURVEY: MENOPAUSE AND THE WORKPLACE: THE FACTS

Menopause can affect women in the workplace in numerous ways. Crushing fatigue can make shift work almost impossible, anxiety that you aren't firing on all cylinders starts to eat away at you and stuffy office environments can trigger hot flushes. Aches and pains can also be a huge hurdle for those with a physically demanding job, and, as I found during my days in general practice, brain fog is a major issue: the ability to stay on top of paperwork, be on the ball in meetings and meet deadlines can be severely hampered by forgetfulness.

In 2021, we surveyed 3,800 perimenopausal and menopausal women about their experiences in the workplace:[232]

- Ninety-nine per cent of respondents said their perimenopausal or menopausal symptoms had led to a negative impact on their careers.
- Fifty-nine per cent had taken time off work due to their symptoms; 18 per cent of these were off more than two months added up over the year.
- Reasons for taking time off included reduced efficiency (45 per cent), poor quality of work (26 per cent) and poor concentration (7 per cent).
- Fifty per cent of those who took at least two months off work resigned or took early retirement.
- Overall, 21 per cent passed on the chance to go for a promotion they would otherwise have considered, 19 per cent reduced hours and 12 per cent resigned.
- Just 5.2 per cent of women who had a sickness certificate issued for time off work had 'menopause' cited on their certificate, while more than a third had 'anxiety' or 'stress' documented.

- Worryingly, 60 per cent of women said their workplace offered no menopause support whatsoever.

These findings speak for themselves. For something half the working population will experience, the lack of support is glaringly obvious. As Anna puts it below – she had to work twice as hard, but even then she was medically retired. Things have to change. Menopausal women are working harder to cover up their symptoms and this simply isn't sustainable.

In 2022, we surveyed over 1,200 menopausal women working in the NHS. Almost half of the respondents (47 per cent) had thought about quitting their jobs as a result of menopausal symptoms. Of those who had started taking HRT, the majority (74 per cent) felt that this had improved their ability to carry on working.[233]

Other research we have undertaken has shown that 74 per cent of women using my free balance app had become more confident talking about menopause in their workplaces and 44 per cent reported that they thought less about resigning or reducing their hours.[234]

This is really important, as around 40 per cent of NHS employees are menopausal women.

CASE STUDY: I HAD TO RETIRE; I'D LOVE TO GET BACK INTO WORK – ANNA'S STORY

'I've always suffered with heavy, painful periods that came with killer mood swings. But, when I was forty-two, I started to experience extreme pain in the middle of my cycle. Around the same time,

I began to have trouble sleeping, and I became very tearful and bad-tempered. Along with feeling very tired, I started to feel a strange sensation on my back, like spiders crawling on my skin. My doctor ordered blood tests but said the results were normal – it wasn't the menopause.

'The following year, I started to have trouble sitting comfortably. My doctor blamed it on my osteoarthritis, and I was so busy working as a ward sister on a dementia ward that I put it down to the physical demands of my job. My symptoms got worse when I started a new job as a senior nurse practitioner in an adult community-health team. It was a sedentary job: I was either sitting at my desk, driving or visiting patients. As well as the pain in my vagina, pelvis and inner thighs, my left hip and knee hurt when I tried to sit.

'My doctor referred me to the pain clinic, and I was prescribed duloxetine and amitriptyline for nerve pain. When these didn't work, I was given gabapentin, then pregabalin and finally fentanyl patches, which made my skin erupt. None of them worked. As a last resort, I was put on morphine tablets, then methadone. I could no longer work full time and I felt like a zombie.

'I was in excruciating pain, especially when my period was due. I felt like something was pushing down between my legs and sitting was a nightmare. I was sent to a neurologist, who did an MRI scan, said everything looked fine and referred me to a gynaecologist. I could hardly walk.

'After another spell of sick leave, I returned to work with a new manager, who was very unsympathetic. I knew that I was on the verge of losing my job, so I decided to get a second opinion – just to buy myself some extra time. I'm glad I did because, after further investigations, I was offered a hysterectomy. This confirmed that I had a cyst on my ovary, fibroids, endometriosis, an enlarged womb and adenomyosis (a condition that causes the lining of the womb – endometrium – to bury deep into the muscular wall of the womb). After the surgery, I woke up pain-free for the first time in six years. It was such a relief, and I honestly believed I was going to be ok. A week later, the pain and burning came back.

'Despite this, I returned to work and tried to pretend that everything was fine. I went to work in the morning, then collapsed at home in the evening. I was absolutely exhausted, not sleeping, in pain and having hot flushes all the time. I looked ten years older and had huge bags under my eyes – but I wasn't going to be beaten because I wanted to keep my job.

'That's when the brain fog started. I was missing things in my diary, but I managed to cover that up – although I had to work harder to make up for it. I also became very anxious. I'd wake up every morning with butterflies in my tummy and the fatigue was so bad that I'd spend weekends doing nothing but trying to catch up on my sleep. I developed pins and needles in my hands and feet and was diagnosed with peripheral neuropathy.

'My symptoms continued to get worse. In 2015, I was diagnosed with tinnitus, pudendal neuralgia [long-term pelvic pain] and vulvodynia [persistent, unexplained pain in the vulva] and I was signed off work. I had three sets of painkilling injections through my vagina into the pudendal nerve in my pelvis. The pain was so horrendous that I didn't go back for any subsequent appointments.

'After that, I lost my job – I was medically retired. I was heartbroken, as I absolutely loved my job. I'd helped so many people and had much more to give. It wasn't just a job – it was a calling; I was proud to say I was a nurse. I was put on antidepressants but only took them for a couple of weeks – they weren't going to help me come to terms with losing my job. Around that time, I found a letter that said I should be put on oestrogen patches and progesterone for twelve months after my hysterectomy, so my GP gave me patches, which helped with the hot flushes for a while.

'As I was still in pain, I was seen by a pelvic-floor physio, who could find nothing wrong. I was told to do pelvic-floor exercises, but they made my pain so much worse. I was seen by another physio, a psychologist and a gynaecologist, who said I didn't have pudendal neuralgia. I was also put on a six-week pain plan, but the physiotherapists wouldn't listen to me when I told them how much the exercises hurt.

'Soon after this, I moved to Scotland and changed to a new doctor, who told me I had to come off HRT as I had been on it for two years and "didn't need it any more". But I was a mess without HRT. I had hot flushes, I was leaving the hob on, my memory was mush – I thought I had early-onset dementia. I didn't feel safe, and I was more exhausted than ever.

'I changed GP and ordered HRT by showing them a repeat prescription from my previous address. I got it, but it didn't work as well as before and I was still having hot flushes. That's when, totally by chance, I saw Dr Louise Newson on TV. I followed her advice and asked for a higher dose of patches. I started sleeping better, the pins and needles in my hands and feet disappeared and the hot flushes stopped. Incredibly, the pain in my hip disappeared and I could lie on my left side again.

'Over the last thirteen years, I've suffered so much, had many procedures, seen so many GPs, consultants, physios – and even a professor. None of them had any answers. But, in the space of six weeks, I've come further, and with better results, than in all that time – and that's all because I happened to turn on the TV.

'The worst thing is that all this could have been prevented. I'm absolutely disgusted that there isn't more menopause information out there, and that we don't have menopause nurses in the NHS, or better workplace policies. So many women and their families are suffering needlessly.

'Fortunately, I'm now feeling more positive about the future. I've just celebrated my fifty-fifth birthday, and I'm finally beginning to get my self-worth and self-esteem back. I'd love to get back to work, so that I can help other people – especially women like me. I feel like this is the beginning of a new life for me, and I'm determined to become the best I can possibly be.'

Menopause and your career: making it work for you

If you are dreading another day at work, please don't struggle in silence. If you are at the point where leaving your job looks like the only option, take a second to think things through; remember what a valuable employee you are and that you have so much left to offer. If work is feeling overwhelming, seek support through whatever channels you can. You should only look to leave a job or career on your own terms.

EXPERT VIEW
Going through the menopause in public life – Baroness Sayeeda Warsi,
Lawyer, author, campaigner and politician

Baroness Warsi is a true trailblazer – but, like so many women, she has struggled with brain fog in the workplace. Here, she describes the impact this has had on her career and the strategies she has put in place to help.

I've always prided myself on my ability to think on my feet and articulate an argument, be it in the courtroom, in the House of Lords or in a studio doing live TV or radio. So when I became perimenopausal when I was forty-six, I found the brain fog that came with it completely overwhelming.

I'd be going into meetings unsure if I would be able to remember the most basic of things, like people's names. I was worried about making a mistake (or as I like to call it, a menopause misstep) in my public life, such as losing my train of thought during a debate in the chamber in the House of Lords, or when being asked a question in a live interview.

Be honest
When you misstep, you worry that those around will interpret your mistake or memory lapse as a sign that you aren't up to the job. This, in itself, can trigger other symptoms, like anxiety or hot flushes.

My advice is to be honest with people around you, both professionally and personally, about what you are going through. Be very specific about the way it manifests, be it brain fog like me or physical symptoms, like hot flushes.

Give colleagues very practical advice on what steps they can take to support you, so you are not having to compensate for other people's reactions.

Preparation is key

Planning ahead can really help with the rush of anxiety that can arise from brain fog.

My brain fog has forced me to be even more organised. I've always been a fairly efficient person, but I used to cram in back-to-back meetings, whereas I now plan my diary several months in advance and schedule in a bit of breathing space between appointments, so I can refocus and prepare for the next one.

I also diarise dedicated preparation time – this can be over a period of weeks if I have a big project or events – so I don't leave anything to the last minute. In the past, I would have been able to walk into a room and give a speech with just a few minutes' prep beforehand. Now, I plan in much more time to prepare.

Take a work timeout

It's really important to take some time out for yourself to exercise or just relax.

Two things that have really helped me are yoga and weight training, particularly in relation to my strength and mobility. I find that because I feel physically stronger, I can cope better with the challenges of work.

I also make sure that I take a chunk of time every year to switch off from work completely. I find that when I come back to work, I feel refreshed and my symptoms are improved.

Timeout #1: Key questions to ask yourself

Give yourself time to sit down and think about the following questions:

- How is the perimenopause or menopause affecting your career?
- What steps have you already taken to address any symptoms you are struggling with?
- Have you spoken to your manager yet?
- What support can your employer offer you?
- What needs to change in the workplace?

I'm perimenopausal or menopausal – what are my rights in the workplace?

In the UK, these are the employee rights for people going through the perimenopause or menopause and experiencing symptoms at work:

- To work in a safe, healthy environment including access to toilets, water, ventilation
- To not be subjected to harassment or discriminated against, either directly or indirectly
- The right to sick pay and annual leave

- The right to request flexible working (usually, if you have worked for more than twenty-six weeks at a company – but some organisations, such as the NHS, now offer the right to request flexible working from day one)
- Protection against unfair dismissal (usually, if you have been employed for more than two years)

I'm menopausal – do I have to tell my manager?

Our health and wellbeing can be very private issues but being open with your employer from the outset will probably help in the long run.

It's also worth checking if your company has a menopause policy (many companies are now putting these in place). If there is one, familiarise yourself with it and ensure you are upholding your end as an employee. This might include being open and honest in conversations with managers or human resources.

How should I go about approaching my manager?

If you are struggling, don't delay. Ask to speak to your direct manager; or, if you feel more comfortable, someone in HR. Give it the time it deserves by asking for a standalone meeting (not just tagging it on to the end of an existing one). You may well find that colleagues have picked up that something isn't quite right, so the request may not come as a surprise to them.

In the same way as your first appointment with a healthcare

professional is your chance to advocate for yourself, this meeting is also key. That's why it's best to make some notes beforehand, so you are clear about what the issues are, what changes are needed in the short term and how you can be supported in the long term. You may also want to check if your manager will be making notes of the conversation, in case you need to refer back to it in the future.

It's worth raising the following at your meeting:

- What proactive steps you have taken yourself to tackle symptoms. Have you spoken to a health professional? If you have been prescribed HRT, have you been advised it may take time for symptoms to settle? Transparency is vital at work while those adjustments take place, and your line managers should be aware that there might be a short-term loss in productivity when you start taking HRT.
- Any changes you have made to your diet and lifestyle that your employer can support you with – for example, a longer lunch break for exercise.
- List the short- and long-term adjustments or changes at work that would benefit you – for example, an altered working pattern, working from home, regular breaks. What about looming deadlines or projects?
- Can you get any further support through work, such as a menopause support group, access to talking therapies like CBT or medical advice through employee-assistance programmes?
- Are you comfortable with colleagues being informed about your menopause? If so, would you rather speak to them yourself, or would you prefer that your manager speaks to them for you?

At the end of the meeting, ask for a copy of what has been agreed, so both sides are clear, and ask for a follow-up meeting in a month's time to discuss how things are going. Remember, your symptoms can change and that means support might need to be altered as time goes on.

EXPERT VIEW
Menopause in the workplace – Liz Earle,
Writer, TV presenter, award-winning entrepreneur and author

Liz Earle is synonymous with wellness. A hugely successful entrepreneur, Liz has been enormously supportive of my work, is very candid about her own menopause experience and is a great advocate for women receiving evidence-based menopause advice and treatment.

In hindsight, I was going through the perimenopause during the most stressful time of my professional career – only no one bothered to tell me!

In my mid-late forties, my business partners and I decided to sell the Liz Earle Beauty Co., which meant enormous pressure workwise, managing legal due diligence, flying back and forth from the United States, endless accountant meetings and audits. All the while, I was juggling life running a busy working farm and my husband and four kids.

I suffered crippling headaches and disturbed sleep but put it all down to stressful times. If only I had known then what I know now, and how my fluctuating levels of oestrogen were such a major factor, I would have started HRT so much sooner and saved a great deal of personal pain – which no doubt caught colleagues and family in the crossfire of my tense and lowered moods, too.

A decade on and menopause awareness in the workplace is increasing.

I am often asked by big companies to speak at corporate events, and it is heartening to see that most requested talk topics are based around improving wellbeing at work. A healthier team produces healthier growth, and firms are wising up to this obvious area of employee support, if only to be more productive and profitable.

I will always include speaking on the perimenopause and menopause to these audiences, as it is such a crucial time for working women – a time when so many feel they simply have to leave work because they feel so dreadful. By educating employers as well as employees, we can all hope to see more changes for the better, at work as well as within wider society.

I am witnessing this already – but much more still needs to be done.

My advice on how to thrive at work during the perimenopause and menopause:

- Become much more aware and knowledgeable of what's happening inside your own body. Knowledge, from trusted sources, is power.
- Download the free balance menopause app and start by tracking your symptoms.
- Have discussions with your GP early on in your journey, so they know what you're thinking, and decide whether or not they're going to be the right doctor for you going forwards. Catch small symptoms such as anxiety or heart palpitations before they turn into depression and night sweats.

- Ask to see a copy of your company's menopause policy. If they don't have one, offer to be involved in writing one.
- Use the word 'menopause' as often as you can to normalise it in the workplace and reduce fear and stigma, in much the same way as has happened with the words 'pregnancy' or 'mental health'.

Advice for employers, managers and colleagues

Too many employers look at menopausal women in their forties and worry they have potentially another twenty years of memory lapses or hot flushes ahead of them. In some cases, they might look for ways to gently move them out of the workplace, while making them think it is their own decision.

It's important not to view menopause as an issue that needs 'fixing'. Instead, see your menopausal employees for what they are: real people who are assets to the smooth running of your organisation. Ask yourself: can you afford to lose their skills and their experience?

That you are reading this today is testament to the fact that you want to support your staff, so let's look at the constructive ways in which you can do this for the benefit of both your employees and your business.

What are your obligations as an employer?

As an employer, you have a duty to ensure the health and safety of all your workers, and to flag any risks and issues that impact them – and this includes the menopause. Once an assessment of risk has been done, you have a responsibility to identify and implement whatever possible measures can be put in place to minimise those risks.

Don't make assumptions about what is needed for an individual, as people's experiences vary greatly. Have open conversations and make plans on a case-by-case basis. The onus is on you as the employer to consider what reasonable adjustments can be made to support the individual.

If a staff member is struggling, you need to evidence what measures are put in place to support them with their performance, absence or conduct.

Do not tolerate bullying or banter regarding the menopause or the symptoms it may cause. A lack of evidence of your supportive measures and acceptance of discriminatory remarks may be grounds for unfair dismissal or discrimination claims.

Although the menopause isn't yet protected specifically under the Equality Act 2010, age, sex and disability discrimination are protected characteristics and many menopause-related claims have been successful on these grounds.

EXPERT VIEW
The £10 billion menopause gap: why businesses can't afford to ignore the menopause any longer – Gaele Lalahy,
Chief Operating Officer of the balance menopause support app

Before taking a mid-life career leap to join balance as chief operating officer in 2021, Gaele had already enjoyed an incredibly successful career in consumer electronics, as board member and head of brand communications and Olympic marketing at Panasonic.

Thanks, in no small part, to Gaele's passion, tenacity and can-do attitude, the balance app has grown exponentially. Since its launch, the app has reached over 1 million people worldwide, helping to change the narrative around the perimenopause and menopause and empowering women with the information they need.

According to the World Economic Forum, if we are to continue at the current rate of progress, it will take 151 years to close the gender gap in economic participation and opportunity.[235] One hundred and fifty-one years for women to close that gap! Take a moment to digest that figure. When diversity and inclusion are rightly a key priority for businesses, we have to do better.

Research by Dr Louise shows a clear correlation between the lack of diagnosis and treatment for perimenopausal and menopausal symptoms and the quality of work experience and career progression. Companies are losing female talent at the peaks of their careers, with a proportion of the workforce lacking the confidence to climb the ladder because of undiagnosed and untreated menopause symptoms.

These issues cannot be ignored any longer.

In 2022, balance calculated the financial impact of the menopause on the UK economy. The cost of women leaving the workforce due to the menopause and the associated costs of rehiring and retraining staff was a staggering £10 billion.[236]

But beyond the financial cost, menopause also impacts diversity. When women miss out on promotion into more senior roles, it impairs the capability for companies to innovate and be more creative.

At balance, we are working with UK organisations such as the NHS, and globally with the likes of Diageo to support a profound cultural and organisational change. Organisations are all at different stages of maturity when it comes to menopause in the workplace. We help break down barriers and upskill workforces through live seminars, courses and employers funding access to our award-winning app for their employees.

The impact is already palpable. Our research shows that 74 per cent of balance app users report they feel more confident to talk about the menopause at work; 40 per cent say they have missed fewer days at work, 68 per cent say their mental health has improved and 1 in 4 (25 per cent) say they are more interested in seeking a promotion.

These results are compelling and we are determined to continue on our mission – because if organisations are a catalyst for better menopause education, and give the tools to their employees to reach fast and appropriate diagnosis and care, we can start to enable women to thrive in the workplace, allow them to claim their seats in top positions, provide much-needed role models for our next generation, reduce the gender pay gap and create a more equal society.

Seems like a worthy mission, doesn't it?

I'm a line manager and one (or more) of my team is menopausal. How can I best help them?

As a line manager, a crucial part of your role is holding supportive one-to-one conversations with your team member/s. These are often the first steps in helping an employee get the help they need and where you can signpost and encourage them to use any internal resources you have within your organisation.

Where to start

Think about how and where the first conversation will take place. Remember, this will probably be a difficult meeting for your employee, so try to offer them a couple of options: it needs to be private, but should that be over a coffee or a walk, say? Or would they prefer the office?

Handle it as a process you will keep coming back to together; perimenopause and menopause vary – they are dynamic and can change over months and years, as new symptoms emerge or treatments begin or evolve.

If your organisation doesn't have a menopause policy, then be the person to get the ball rolling. Raise it with the appropriate people, such as your HR department; or if you work for a smaller business, take it to the owner. If there are no formal systems in place for menopause support, link up a couple of individuals (with their permission) who are going through it, so they can support one another and feel less alone.

Are there any resources you can point your employee in the direction of? NICE guidelines, balance app, any company materials (see Expert View, p. 340)?

CASE STUDY: I'M BUILDING A NEW BUSINESS AND A NEW CAREER – LAURA'S STORY

With her first child leaving for university and her two younger children growing up fast, Laura was on the cusp of making some changes in her life when menopause symptoms started. Her experience is far from unusual; many women who come to the clinic find themselves in similar situations.

'Food has always been my passion. Before I had children, I had my own catering business, but after having three kids in five years it became impossible to do the two, so I left catering and took a term-time job in a local secondary school as an administrator.

'The job was part-time, but I found the organisational skills I'd developed when running my business really came into their own in my new role, and I was promoted to increasingly senior roles over the years. A good school thrives on good organisation, and a lot of plate-spinning. My first head teacher used to call me the oracle because I could remember the name of every pupil – no mean feat when you work in a school with hundreds of children.

'I really enjoyed my job, but in the back of my mind, I saw the point where my kids reached their teens and started to go off out in the world as the time when I would go back to my first career. As they got older, I felt I was on the cusp of "my time", where I could get back out there.

'I was forty-five and my eldest daughter had just left for university when what I realise now was perimenopause hit. I was teary, I was forgetful and just really, really tired. I could barely keep my eyes open in meetings sometimes.

'At home I was a bit of a nightmare (my two youngest children bore the brunt of a lot of my miserable moods), but by far the biggest impact was on my working life.

'My most important role was overseeing school exams. Remember how nervous you feel the night before an exam? Well, it felt like I was taking on the worries of whole year groups of children, making sure everything ran smoothly. The fact that one mistake on the exam schedule could have a huge impact on the lives of young people always weighed heavy on me, but this particular year the stress was just insurmountable.

'I would check, re-check and check everything. I put Post-it notes everywhere – by my computer, in my diary, even on the back of my office door. I was so tired that it just felt I had absolutely nothing in the tank.

'At work, we were a close-knit team, so it didn't take long for someone to ask what was wrong with me. One day, a colleague who had become a good friend over the years approached me in the corridor and asked for a quiet word. She explained that she'd noticed I'd been quite flustered and forgetful in recent months and wondered if everything was ok at home.

'God, I was so embarrassed. I was very brusque with her and said something along the lines of minding her own business. But when I got back to my desk, there were tears in my eyes – because I knew, deep down, she was right.

'I tried to focus on my work, but I couldn't shake the feeling that others were watching me, scrutinising my work. I took my colleague's concern for criticism and, as the weeks went on, I became increasingly worried about my job and my mental health really declined. The feeling that I couldn't do my job got worse, to the point where I felt like I had no choice but to leave – that I was unemployable.

'I ended up confiding in my older sister, who was the first person to mention the "menopause" word to me. The more research I did, the more I realised I was probably perimenopausal (I was still having periods at that time). Asking for help isn't really "me", but my sister convinced me to go to my doctor and talk to them about HRT. I did preparation before the appointment – made a list of my symptoms, had a copy of the NICE menopause guidelines – and I left the surgery with a prescription the same day. It took a few months, but the change since I started HRT has been incredible.

'I was pretty candid with colleagues when I started HRT. I told them it might take a few months to get back on to an even keel, and everyone was so supportive. I think having that good working relationship helped me be more upfront, and I do wonder how easy it is for other women in other industries to do the same; friends of mine have had the most terrible time trying to speak to their bosses about what they are going through.

'COVID-19 lockdown re-ignited my love for cooking, and I've since started a monthly supper club. It's early days, but the reviews from customers and repeat bookings have given me such a huge confidence boost that I'm back to my best, and I'm seriously considering taking the leap and leaving my school job in the next year. I know that without HRT I would never have had the energy, confidence or get-up-and-go to try something new.

'It really feels like it's my time.'

Company CEO? Here's what you can do

Addressing the menopause shouldn't be an optional extra; it needs to be an integral part of looking after your workforce as an inclusive employer. So what does good menopause support look like? It involves some – or ideally all – of the following:

- A robust menopause policy that means more than simply another file gathering dust on the shelf
- Providing menopause education for all staff – training managers in the impact it can have at work and how to

support employees (but this doesn't end with managers – your whole workforce should be given information on the common symptoms so they can spot them in colleagues)

- Peer-support systems, such as a menopause support group, including menopause champions, mentors for those experiencing symptoms, role models for one-to-one support and advice to managers
- Specialist training for HR and occupational-health staff
- Access to menopause specialist clinics, if appropriate

Why an open menopause culture is key

The suggestions above are all well and good, but processes, policies and support groups mean nothing in isolation.

As a CEO, you should be setting the example by normalising conversation about the menopause. You can help spread the message that help and effective treatments are out there, and facilitate people accessing accurate information and medical help.

How can I support my colleagues who are experiencing perimenopausal or menopausal symptoms?

This is not just an issue for women or HR staff. Those who don't go through the menopause will be indirectly affected via partners, mothers, sisters, friends or work colleagues. So whoever you are, here are some tips on how to support your colleagues:

- Learn a bit about the basics to show you're making an effort to understand and attend any menopause-education sessions at work.
- Be open to having a conversation if it crops up, and brave enough to initiate one if it's relevant.
- Get comfortable with saying the words 'periods', 'perimenopause' and 'menopause'. Try saying them aloud right now. See? It's easy!
- Recognise that the effects can start years before periods stop and can cause an array of physical and psychological symptoms, even to the point where someone can seem completely unlike their usual self, and they may or may not themselves realise what's going on.
- Know that HRT is safe and effective for the majority who need it, and it's available on the NHS.
- Familiarise yourself with any help that's available within your organisation when being an ally to a colleague, such as the menopause policy key features and types of support available.

13

Looking to the Future

Public speaking isn't everyone's cup of tea.

For many, the idea of getting up in front of a group of complete strangers, even for a few brief minutes, is enough to fill them with dread. On the other hand, some people positively thrive on it, running on adrenaline while sharing information and anecdotes.

Up until a few years ago, I was firmly in the former camp. Public speaking was the last thing I could see myself doing on a regular basis.

Why?

I was bullied at school. What should have been some of the happiest years of my life were tinged with painful memories of feeling like the odd one out, worried about showing my true self in case people would laugh at or tease me.

Losing my beloved father at a young age had a lasting impact, too. I was so confident when I had two parents and my world was shattered when he died. I missed him terribly; I felt so cheated that he had died so young, and it took many years before

I could go through an entire day without being sad and thinking about him. Even now, I wonder how different I would be if I had grown up with a father.

The feeling that I wasn't quite good enough lingered well into my university years and beyond, into my medical career. I remember going up on stage to collect my medical degree during my graduation – the all-too-familiar knot in my stomach, my hands clammy as I held on to my scroll and mortar board for dear life. Outwardly, I seemed fine, but inwardly I told myself that I wasn't deserving of the accolade, despite having worked my socks off. That I wasn't as good as my classmates, though my results suggested otherwise. I thought to myself: what on earth was I thinking getting up there on stage?

That was back in the 1990s, and what I thought were 'just nerves' I now know to be imposter syndrome. Even when I passed my Membership of the Royal College of General Practitioners (MRCGP) exam with distinction, I told others that I was just lucky. I have always doubted my ability, and today I still worry about the things I have not achieved, rather than the many I have accomplished.

It's the same feeling I had when I sat at the kitchen table with my husband, Paul, writing a list of the pros and cons of going it alone to start my own clinic, leaving my safe job as a GP and the NHS.

Starting a private clinic felt like a necessity (I could not open an NHS menopause clinic as there was no funding or interest in NHS hospitals and clinics near me). As I outlined at the start of this book, it never was, nor will it ever be about money for me. My ambition to open the clinic and develop both the website and the balance app were driven by a desire to reach as many people as possible, giving them access to evidence-based information, enabling them to make decisions about the treatment that is right for them. It would have been easy to carry on living in my own bubble, but the stories I heard from women sitting in my consulting room and the accounts I interacted with on social media gave me the push I needed to leave my GP job to try to improve things by working differently.

In addition, my personal experience of not having had access to help for my own symptoms meant that doing nothing was simply not an option for me. And knowing that so many women needed things to change gave me the impetus to cast doubts aside and forge ahead on my own; and it remains my main motivation to this day.

So that's why, when I stood up at a lectern in September 2022 and gave a keynote speech at a two-day conference for female clinicians, it felt like things were coming full circle. Buoyed by my experiences, I have grown in confidence and had given numerous presentations before – but this time it was different. It was the first time my team and I, along with the Women in Medicine International Network, had organised a conference on the theme of creating an environment for women to thrive in medicine.

It was incredible, informative and inspiring – and being among such a fantastic group of people gave me great hope for the future. So many women in healthcare and beyond gave their time to speak and, in their presence, I felt confident, empowered and excited about what can be in achieved in the coming years. I'm not a lone voice, but in the company of so many people – men, as well as women – who are also fighting to make things better.

At the conference, many spoke about the twin challenges of working in healthcare and coping with their own menopause. In addition, Baroness Warsi (see Expert View, p. 332) talked about the menopause and public life; journalist and menopause activist Kate Muir (we will be hearing more from Kate in a moment) spoke powerfully about the challenges of menopause in the workplace; and Liz Earle MBE (see Expert View, p. 337) spoke about the importance of looking after ourselves as we become more successful and have less time.

I do let myself acknowledge the successes that keep menopause in the public psyche – launching a charity, the two-millionth download of my podcast or being profiled in national newspapers – not out of a sense of ego, but in reflecting on how the menopause conversation has changed in the last decade. But to me, the moments most worthy of celebration are when I receive a message from a woman – whether it is an email from someone in my direct care or someone on the other side of the world connecting through social media – to tell me I have made a difference.

In my clinic, we share feedback from our patients weekly because it reminds us of why we do what we do.

And yes, being among that group of inspiring women at our conference was proof of progress. But we cannot afford to rest on our laurels.

Recent HRT supply issues prove a growing awareness that help is out there, but the fact remains that too few women who would stand to benefit from transformative treatment like HRT are able to access it, especially in areas of deprivation. Many are still facing multiple appointments before getting the help they need, and socioeconomic status and ethnicity present additional major barriers to treatment: one study found the overall prescribing rate of HRT was 29 per cent lower in English GP practices in the most deprived areas compared with the most affluent.[237] This has to change.

Access to treatment should be based on need, not economic status, skin colour or postcode.

EXPERT VIEW
Why I became a menopause activist – Kate Muir,
Author and journalist

Kate is an incredible force of nature – first as a patient, then as an ally in spreading awareness and finally as a friend.

I became a menopause activist in Dr Louise Newson's consulting room. She sorted out my HRT, then told me a story that changed my life, her life and – eventually – millions of women's lives.

Louise told me about a woman in her forties who had been diagnosed with 'treatment-resistant depression'. Antidepressants had no effect on her anxiety, fear of leaving the house and inability to feel joy. She left her job and was also suffering from painful genitourinary symptoms and hot flushes.

No one spotted the perimenopausal clues. Instead, her NHS consultant sent her for ECT – electro-convulsive therapy – as an outpatient at a psychiatric facility. Between 70 and 100 volts of electricity were fired through her head, over twelve sessions.

The woman struggled for years afterwards, barely leaving her armchair, until she began googling 'hormonal depression' and found ut about Louise's clinic. Because she was agoraphobic, her husband had to drive her to the appointment. She got HRT, and a week later walked her dog for the first time in seven years. The depression was gone.

I was so incensed by that story that I went from patient to investigative journalist within the space of a few minutes. 'I can't let that happen to anyone else,' I said, ringing a friend on the way home. 'We're going to make a documentary about the menopause,' I added. 'But you've never made a documentary before,' she said.

Three years later, and not without a struggle, I am now a television producer and have created two Channel 4 menopause documentaries, presented by Davina McCall. Louise appeared as our medical expert in the first film, and audiences for both reached almost 6 million. In the year after the first broadcast, HRT prescriptions went up by half a million.

Newspapers called it 'The Davina Effect', as the menopause taboo was busted. But it was really 'The Louise Newson Effect' that started it all. What Louise brings to the increasingly gladiatorial menopause arena is razor-sharp, triple-checked scientific knowledge of the latest advances, and a deep empathy for her patients.

It helps that we're both women of menopausal age ourselves, living the dream – or watching the nightmare, when women are left without treatment.

I sought out private HRT (after an NHS refusal) when my memory started to fail. As the daughter of Alzheimer's, that terrified me. I was writing a shopping list, thinking, 'Must shave my legs,' and wrote down the word 'shaver'. Then I thought, 'There's another word for that thing,' panicking. It took me half an hour to remember the word 'razor'.

Once I started HRT, my memory came zinging back, and my heart palpitations and night sweats stopped within days. I became evangelical about understanding and explaining the science behind the new, safer body-identical HRT to as many women as possible, and the latest studies showing it does not increase the risk of breast cancer.[238]

Researching my own book, Everything You Need to Know About the Menopause (but were too afraid to ask), I delved deep into years of research showing the positive effect of oestrogen (and testosterone) replacement on osteoporosis, type 2 diabetes, heart disease and dementia. Now I'm working alongside Louise to get that message of lifelong health improvement on HRT out there. It's a huge gift waiting for women. And I want them to have the second chance I've been given.

My final message to you

....

When I started writing this book, I envisaged it as a trusted resource that everyone – whether menopausal or not – could reach for and be able to read facts in a clear, easily accessible way.

And I now want to end it with a message to you.

Whatever your reasons for picking up this book, thank you. Every woman, regardless of background, deserves a good and healthy menopause. And that starts with awareness, to which I hope this book contributes.

To those of you in government roles, or who have the crucial job of educating our next generation: good menopause care begins with access to good menopause education. We can't afford to let future generations of women suffer in silence. The menopause needs to be discussed openly in classrooms, lecture theatres and tutorial groups.

To those of you in management roles, whether you look after a small team or are responsible for the running of a large corporation: it's not enough to say you are menopause-friendly; you have to practise what you preach. Be a role model in your organisation: listen, use the M-word in meetings; normalise it. Signpost women to the right medical help, so they can continue working in roles that they can excel at. So many of us spend so much of our lives at work that it is imperative it is a space where we feel supported and valued.

To the partners, siblings, friends and other loved ones of those going through the perimenopause and menopause: talking is healthy, but you can also be agents of action. If you feel your loved one is struggling, gently suggest that they might benefit from speaking to a healthcare professional.

To children and teenagers: I know you are probably a bit

worried about your mum, step-mum or a relative if you've noticed some changes in their behaviour recently. Please be reassured that they love you as much as they always have but are going through a difficult time. It's so important you try to talk to them, or another adult, about how you are feeling. Try to encourage them to access help and treatment. My daughters and I have been there and come out the other side – and that's involved lots of talking.

To healthcare professionals: I've met many peers who are doing incredible work in advancing women's health, but we all know improvements are needed. You can develop your knowledge by taking my free Confidence in the Menopause course for healthcare professionals, which has been downloaded more than 30,000 times. Look at the latest evidence and hold shared decision making at the heart of everything you do. All women deserve the time and the opportunity to sit down and discuss their symptoms, treatment options, medical history and personal preferences with a healthcare professional.

And finally, to those of you who are going through the perimenopause and menopause right now: you may feel lonely, angry, confused, worried or a complete mixture of emotions. This is normal, but it doesn't have to be like this for ever. You can absolutely thrive during this time, but you need to be kind to yourself and ask for the help and treatment that are right for you. Keep this book and dip in whenever you need answers and advice. Use the resources listed on pp. 357–360. Talk to friends, family, work colleagues and health professionals.

Remember, this is a life event that *every woman* will go through – 47 million globally just this year.[239]

Above all, remember you are not alone.

Resources

Menopause information and support

- Balance app, balance-menopause.com/balance-app
- Balance website, free menopause information and advice, balance-menopause.com
- Dr Louise Newson Podcast, balance-menopause.com/type /podcast
- International Menopause Society, imsociety.org
- Newson Health Menopause and Wellbeing Centre, newson-health.co.uk
- The Menopause Charity, themenopausecharity.org

Menopause guidelines

- National Institute for Health and Care Excellence (NICE), Menopause: Diagnosis and management guideline, nice.org.uk/guidance/ng23
- NICE, POI guideline, nice.org.uk/guidance/ng23/ifp/chapter /Premature-menopause-premature-ovarian-insufficiency

Cardiovascular health

....

- British Heart Foundation, Manage your Blood Pressure at Home guide, bhf.org.uk

Early menopause and POI

....

- Daisy Network, POI charity, daisynetwork.org
- Trekstock, young adult cancer support, trekstock.com

Exercise

....

- Parkrun, free community walks and runs worldwide, parkrun.com
- The Body Coach, Joe Wicks, thebodycoach.com
- This Girl Can, taster classes, thisgirlcanclasses.co.uk/this-girl-can-classes

Inclusive resources

....

- People Arise Now, peoplearisenow.org, community-support organisation, based in London, peoplerisenow.org
- Keep the Drums Lose the Knife, community-interest

organisation, which aims to stamp out all forms of violence against women and children, with a focus on ending FGM, keepthedrumsandlosetheknife.org

- The Sophia Forum, sophiaforum.net, organisation that promotes and advocates for the rights, health, welfare and dignity of women living with HIV, sophiaforum.net

Mental health and wellbeing

- British Association of Mindfulness-Based Approaches (BAMBA), searchable list of mindfulness teachers, bamba.org.uk/teachersearch
- CBT register for the UK and Ireland, cbtregisteruk.com
- Headspace, meditation app, headspace.com
- Liz Earle Wellbeing, writer, TV presenter, author and entrepreneur, lizearlewellbeing.com

Nutrition

- Emma Ellice Flint, clinical nutritionist, emmasnutrition.com
- Dr Sally Norton, weight management expert and consultant surgeon, drsallynorton.com
- The Doctor's Kitchen, blog and podcast from Dr Rupy Aujla, thedoctorskitchen.com
- Zoe Health Study, health-study.joinzoe.com

Postnatal depression (PND)

- PANDAS Foundation, PND awareness and support, pandas-foundation.org.uk.

Premenstrual syndrome (PMS) and premenstrual dysphoric disorder (PMDD)

- Association for Premenstrual Syndrome (NAPS), Daily Record of Severity of Problems, pms.org.uk/support/menstrual-diary
- International Association for Premenstrual Disorders, symptom tracker, iapmd.org/symptomtracker

Resources for healthcare professionals

- The Newson Health Menopause Society, a multidisciplinary team of healthcare professionals and experts passionate about improving and understanding women's hormone health, nhmenopausesociety.org
- Women in Medicine International Network, networking and information sharing network, wimin.org

References

Chapter 1

1. Rosato, E., Sciarra, F., Anastasiadou, E., Lenzi, A., Venneri, M. A. (2022), 'Revisiting the physiological role of androgens in women', *Expert Review of Endocrinology & Metabolism*, doi: 10.1080/17446651.2022.2144834. Epub ahead of print. PMID: 36352537

2. Takeda, T. (2022), 'Premenstrual disorders: Premenstrual syndrome and premenstrual dysphoric disorder', *Journal of Obstetrics and Gynaecology Research*, Advance online publication. https://doi.org/10.1111/jog.15484

3. Ryu, A., Kim, T. H. (2015), 'Premenstrual syndrome: A mini review', *Maturitas*, 82 (4), pp. 436–40. https://doi.org/10.1016/j.maturitas.2015.08.010

4. NHS.uk (2018), 'Feeling depressed after childbirth', https://www.nhs.uk/conditions/baby/support-and-services/feeling-depressed-after-childbirth

Chapter 2

5. British Fertility Society, 'At what age does fertility begin to decrease?', https://www.britishfertilitysociety.org.uk/fei/at-what-age-does-fertility-begin-to-decrease

6. Luine, V., Frankfurt M. (2013), 'Interactions between estradiol, BDNF and dendritic spines in promoting memory', *Neuroscience*, 3 239, pp. 34–45. doi: 10.1016/j.neuroscience.2012.10.019

7. Celec, P., Ostatníková, D., Hodosy, J. (2015), 'On the effects of testosterone on brain behavioral functions', *Frontiers of Neuroscience*. doi: 10.3389/fnins.2015.00012

8. NHS.uk (2021), 'Salt: the facts' https://www.nhs.uk/live-well/eat-well/food-types/salt-nutrition/#

9. Yung, J. A., Fuseini, H., Newcomb, D. C. (2018), 'Hormones, sex, and asthma', *Annals of Allergy, Asthma & Immunology*, 120 (5). pp. 488–94. doi: 10.1016/j.anai.2018.01.016

10. Triebner, K. et al. (2017), 'Menopause is associated with accelerated lung function decline', *American Journal of Respiratory and Critical Care Medicine*, 195 (8), pp. 1058–65. doi:10.1164/rccm.201605-0968OC

11. Terauchi, M., Odai, T., Hirose, A., Kato, K., Akiyoshi, M., Masuda, M., Tsunoda, R., Fushiki, H., Miyasaka, N. (2018), 'Dizziness in peri- and postmenopausal women is associated with anxiety: a cross-sectional study', *BioPsychoSocial Medicine*, doi: 10.1186/s13030-018-0140-1

12. Peck, T. et al. (2017), 'Dry eye syndrome in menopause and perimeno-pausal age group', *Journal of Mid-life Health*, 8(2), pp. 51–4. doi:10.4103/jmh.JMH_41_17

13. Dutt, P., Chaudhary, S., Kumar, P. (2013), 'Oral health and menopause: a comprehensive review on current knowledge and associated dental management', *Annals of Medical and Health Sciences Research*, 3(3) pp. 320–3, doi: 10.4103/2141-9248.117926

14. Suri, V., Suri, V. (2014), 'Menopause and oral health', *Journal of Mid-life Health*, 5 (3), pp. 115–20, doi:10.4103/0976-7800.141187

15. Delhez, A., Lefebvre, P., Péqueux, C., Malgrange, B., Delacroix, L. (2020), 'Auditory function and dysfunction: estrogen makes a difference', *Cellular and Molecular Life Sciences*, 77 (4) pp. 619–35. doi: 10.1007/s00018-019-03295-y

16. Carpenter, J. S., Sheng, Y., Pike, C., Elomba, C. D., Alwine, J. S., Chen, C. X., Tisdale, J. E. (2022), 'Correlates of palpitations during menopause: A scoping review', *Womens Health*, doi: 10.1177/17455057221112267

17. Infantino, M. (2008), 'The prevalence and pattern of gastroesophageal reflux symptoms in perimenopausal and menopausal women', *Journal of the American Academy of Nurse Practitioners*, 20 (5), pp. 266–72, https://doi.org/10.1111/j.1745-7599.2008.00316.x

18. Deecher, D. C., Dorries, K. (2007), 'Understanding the pathophysiology of vasomotor symptoms (hot flushes and night sweats) that occur in peri-menopause, menopause, and postmenopause life stages', *Archives of Women's Mental Health*, 10 (6) pp. 247–57. doi.org/10.1007/s00737-007-0209-5

19. Hussain, S. M., Cicuttini, F. M., Alyousef, B., Wang, Y. (2018), 'Female hormonal factors and osteoarthritis of the knee, hip and hand: a narrative review', *Climacteric*, 21(2), pp. 132–9. doi: 10.1080/13697137.2017.1421926

20. Dennison, E. M. (2022), 'Osteoarthritis: The importance of hormonal status in midlife women', *Maturitas*, 165, pp. 8–11. doi: 10.1016/j.maturitas.2022.07.002

21. Islam, R. M., Bell, R. J., Green, S., Page, M. J., Davis, S. R. (2019), 'Safety and efficacy of testosterone for women: a systematic review and meta-analysis of randomised controlled trial data', *Lancet Diabetes Endocrinology*, 7 (10), pp. 754–66. doi: 10.1016/S2213-8587(19)30189-5

22. Hipolito Rodrigues, M. A., Maitrot-Mantelet, L., Plu-Bureau, G., Gompel, A. (2018), 'Migraine, hormones and the menopausal transition', *Climacteric*, 21 (3), pp. 256–66. doi: 10.1080/13697137.2018.1439914

23. Perry, S., Shaw, C., Assassa, P. et al. (2000), 'Leicestershire MRC Incontinence Study Team. An epidemiological study to establish the prevalence of urinary symptoms and felt need in the community: the Leicestershire MRC Incontinence Study', *Journal of Public Health Medicine*, 22 (3): pp. 427–34, doi.org/10.1093/pubmed/22.3.427

24. Luthje, P., Browner, H., Ramos, N. L. et al. (2013), 'Estrogen supports urothelial defense mechanisms', *Science Translational Medicine*, 5 (190); 190ra80 doi:10.1126/scitranslmed.3005574

25. Beerepoot, M. A. et al. (2013), 'Non-antibiotic prophylaxis for recurrent UTI; a systematic review and meta-analysis of RCTs, *Journal of Urology*, 190 (6), pp. 1981–9, doi:10.1016/j.juro.2013.04.142

26. Krychman, M., Graham, S., Bernick, B., Mirkin, S., Kingsberg, S. A. (2017), 'The women's EMPOWER survey: women's knowledge and awareness of treatment options for vulvar and vaginal atrophy remains inadequate', *Journal of Sexual Medicine*, 14 (3), pp. 425–33. doi: 10.1016/j.jsxm.2017.01.011

27. Portman, D. J., Gass, M. L. (2014), 'Genitourinary syndrome of menopause: new terminology for vulvovaginal atrophy from the International Society for the Study of Women's Sexual Health and the North American Menopause Society,' *Menopause*, 21 (10), pp. 1063–8. doi: 10.1097/GME.0000000000000329

Chapter 3

28. Office for National Statistics (2015), 'Victory in Europe Day: How World War II changed the UK', https://www.ons.gov.uk/peoplepopulationandcommunity/birthsdeathsandmarriages/articles/victoryineuropedayhowworldwariichangedtheuk/2015-05-08

29. Office for National Statistics (2022), 'Past and projected period and cohort life tables: 2020-based, UK, 1981 to 2070', https://www.ons.gov.uk/peoplepopulationandcommunity/birthsdeathsandmarriages/lifeexpectancies/bulletins/pastandprojecteddatafromtheperiodandcohortlifetables/2020baseduk1981to2070

30. Cramer, D. W., Xu, H., Harlow, B. L. (1995), 'Family history as a predictor of early menopause', *Fertility and Sterility*, 64(4), pp. 740–5, doi:10.1016/s0015-0282(16)57849-2

31. Ibid.

32. Rees, M. (1995) 'The age of menarche', *ORGYN: Organon's Magazine on Women and Health*, 4, pp. 2–4

33. All-Party Parliamentary Group on Menopause (2022), Inquiry to assess the impacts of menopause and the case for policy reform: concluding report, https://menopause-appg.co.uk/wp-content/uploads/2022/10/APPG-Menopause-Inquiry-Concluding-Report-12.10.22-1.pdf

Chapter 4

34. National Institute for Health and Care Excellence (NICE) (2015), 'Menopause: diagnosis and management', www.nice.org.uk/guidance/ng23

35. Gambacciani, M. et al. (2019), 'Hormone replacement therapy and prevention of chronic conditions', *Climacteric*, 22 (3), pp. 303–06. doi:10.1080/13697137.2018.1551347

36. Zhu L., Jiang X., Sun Y., Shu W., (2016), 'Effect of hormone therapy on the risk of bone fractures: a systematic review and meta-analysis of randomized controlled trials', *Menopause*, 23(4), pp. 461–70. doi: 10.1097/GME.0000000000000519

37. Trémollieres F. (2019), 'Assessment and hormonal management of osteoporosis', *Climacteric*, 22 (2), pp. 122–6, doi: 10.1080/13697137.2018.1555582

38. El Khoudary, S. R. et al. (2020), 'Menopause transition and cardiovascular disease risk: implications for timing of early prevention: a scientific statement from the American Heart Association', *Circulation*, 142 (25), e506–32. doi:10.1161/CIR.0000000000000912

39. Boardman, H. et al. (2015), 'Hormone therapy for preventing cardiovascular disease in post-menopausal women', *Cochrane database of systematic reviews*, doi:10.1002/14651858.CD002229.pub4

40. Lobo, R. A. et al. (2016), 'Back to the future: Hormone replacement therapy as part of a prevention strategy for women at the onset of menopause', *Atherosclerosis*, 254 (2016): 282–90. doi:10.1016/j.atherosclerosis.2016.10.005

41. Anand S. S. et al. (2008), 'INTERHEART Investigators. Risk factors for myocardial infarction in women and men: insights from the INTERHEART study', *European Heart Journal*, 29 (7), pp. 932–40. doi: 10.1093/eurheartj/ehn018. Epub 2008 Mar 10. PMID: 18334475

42. Thurston, R. C. et al. (2021), 'Menopausal vasomotor symptoms and risk of incident cardiovascular disease events in SWAN', *Journal of the American Heart Association*, 10 (3), e017416. doi:10.1161/JAHA.120.017416

43. Ley, S. H. et al. (2017), 'Duration of reproductive life span, age at menarche, and age at menopause are associated with risk of cardiovascular disease in women', *Journal of the American Heart Association*, 6 (11), doi:10.1161/JAHA.117.006713

44. Harvey, R. E., Coffman, K. E., Miller, V. M. (2015), 'Women-specific factors to consider in risk, diagnosis and treatment of cardiovascular disease', *Womens Health*, 11 (2), pp. 239–57. doi: 10.2217/whe.14.64. PMID: 25776297; PMCID: PMC4386625

45. Newson, L. (2018), 'Menopause and cardiovascular disease', *Post Reproductive Health*, 24 (1), pp. 44–9. doi: 10.1177/2053369117749675

46. Xiang, D. et al. (2021), 'Protective effects of estrogen on cardiovascular disease mediated by oxidative stress', *Oxidative Medicine and Cellular Longevity*, doi:10.1155/2021/5523516

47. Lobo, R. A. (1990), 'Cardiovascular implications of estrogen replacement therapy', *Obstetrics and Gynecology*, doi: 10.1016/0020-7292(90)90539-w

48. Maclaran K., Stevenson J. C. (2012), 'Primary prevention of cardiovascular disease with HRT', *Womens Health*, 8 (1) pp. 63–74. doi: 10.2217/whe.11.87

49. Lobo, R. A., Pickar, J. H., Stevenson, J. C., Mack, W. J., Hodis, H. N. (2016), 'Back to the future: Hormone replacement therapy as part of a prevention strategy for women at the onset of menopause', *Atherosclerosis*, 254: pp. 282–90. doi: 10.1016/j.atherosclerosis.2016.10.005

50. Maruthur, N. M., Wang, N. Y., Appel, L. J. (2009), 'Lifestyle interventions reduce coronary heart disease risk: results from the PREMIER Trial', *Circulation*, 119 (15) pp. 2026–31. doi: 10.1161/CIRCULATIONAHA.108.80949

51. Manson, J. E., Aragaki, A. K., Rossouw, J. E., et al. (2015), 'Menopausal hormone therapy and long-term all-cause and cause-specific mortality: The Women's Health Initiative randomized trials', *JAMA*, 318 (10), pp. 927–38. doi:10.1001/jama.2017.11217

52. Boardman H. M., Hartley, L., Eisinga, A., Main, C., Roqué i Figuls, M., Bonfill Cosp, X., Gabriel Sanchez, R., Knight, B. (2015), 'Hormone therapy for preventing cardiovascular disease in post-menopausal women', *Cochrane Database of Systemic Reviews*, 10 (3):CD002229. doi: 10.1002/14651858.CD002229.pub4

53. Salpeter, S. R., Cheng, J., Thabane, L., Buckley, N. S., Salpeter, E. E. (2009), 'Bayesian meta-analysis of hormone therapy and mortality in younger postmenopausal women', *American Journal of Medicine*, 122 (11):1016-1022.e1. doi: 10.1016/j.amjmed.2009.05.021

54. El Khoudary, S. R. et al. (2020), 'Menopause transition and cardiovascular disease risk: implications for timing of early prevention: a scientific statement from the American Heart Association', *Circulation*, 142 (25), e506-e532. doi:10.1161/CIR.0000000000000912

55. NHS.uk (2021), 'Blood pressure test', www.nhs.uk/conditions/blood-pressure-test

56. Nappi, R. E., Chedraui, P., Lambrinoudaki, I., Simoncini, T. (2022), 'Menopause: a cardiometabolic transition', *Lancet Diabetes and Endocrinology*, 10 (6), pp. 442–56. doi.org/10.1016/S2213-8587(22)00076-6

57. Slopien, R. et al. (2018), 'Menopause and diabetes: EMAS clinical guide', *Maturitas*, doi: 10.1016/j.maturitas.2018.08.009

58. Grodstein, F., Newcomb, P. A., Stampfer, M. J. (1999), 'Postmenopausal hormone therapy and the risk of colorectal cancer: a review and meta-analysis', *American Journal of Medicine*, 106(5) pp. 574–82. doi: 10.1016/s0002-9343(99)00063-7

59. Manson, J. E. et al. (2013), 'Menopausal hormone therapy and health outcomes during the intervention and extended poststopping phases of the Women's Health Initiative randomized trials', *JAMA*, 310 (13), pp. 1353–68. doi:10.1001/jama.2013.278040

60. Akter, N., Kulinskaya, E., Steel, N., Bakbergenuly, I. (2022), 'The effect of hormone replacement therapy on the survival of UK women: a retrospective cohort study 1984-2017', *BJOG*, 129 (6):994–1003. doi:10.1111/1471-0528.17008

61. Trenti, A. et al. (2018), 'Estrogen, angiogenesis, immunity and cell metabolism: solving the puzzle', *International Journal of Molecular Sciences*, 19 (3), doi:10.3390/ijms19030859

62. Kim, Y. J. et al. (2021), 'Association between menopausal hormone therapy and risk of neurodegenerative diseases: Implications for precision hormone therapy', *Alzheimer's and Dementia*, 7 (1) e12174, doi:10.1002/trc2.12174

63. Jett S. et al. (2022), 'Endogenous and exogenous estrogen exposures: how women's reproductive health can drive brain aging and inform alzheimer's prevention', *Frontiers in Aging Neuroscience*, doi:10.3389/fnagi.2022.831807

64. Jett S. et al. (2022) 'Ovarian steroid hormones: a long overlooked but critical contributor to brain aging and Alzheimer's disease', *Frontiers in*

Aging Neuroscience, doi:10.3389/fnagi.2022.948219

65. Kim, Y. J. et al. (2021), 'Association between menopausal hormone therapy and risk of neurodegenerative diseases: Implications for precision hormone therapy', *Alzheimer's and Dementia,* 7 (1) e12174, doi:10.1002/trc2.12174

66. Davey, D. A. (2018), 'Menopausal hormone therapy: a better and safer future', *Climacteric,* 21 (5), pp. 454–61, doi: 10.1080/13697137.2018.1439915

67. Office for National Statistics, 'Births in England and Wales: 2020', https://www.ons.gov.uk/peoplepopulationandcommunity/birthsdeathsand-marriages/livebirths/bulletins/birthsummarytablesenglandandwales/2020

68. Langer, R. D., Hodis, H. N., Lobo, R. A., Allison, M. A. (2021), 'Hormone replacement therapy – where are we now?', *Climacteric,* 24 (1), pp. 3–10. doi: 10.1080/13697137.2020.1851183

69. Vinogradova, Y., Coupland, C., Hippisley-Cox, J. (2019), 'Use of hormone replacement therapy and risk of venous thromboembolism: nested case-control studies using the QResearch and CPRD databases', *British Medical Journal,* 364:k4810. doi: 10.1136/bmj.k4810. Erratum in: *BMJ.* 2019 Jan 15;364:l162

70. Straczek, C., Oger, E., Yon de Jonage-Canonico, M. B., Plu-Bureau, G., Conard, J., Meyer, G., Alhenc-Gelas, M., Lévesque, H., Trillot, N., Barrellier, M. T., Wahl, D., Emmerich, J., Scarabin, P. Y. (2005), 'Estrogen and thrombo-embolism risk (ESTHER) study group. Prothrombotic mutations, hormone therapy, and venous thromboembolism among postmenopausal women: impact of the route of estrogen administration', *Circulation,* 112(22):3495–500. doi: 10.1161/CIRCULATIONAHA.105.565556

71. Tan D.A., Dayu A.R.B. (2022), 'Menopausal hormone therapy: why we should no longer be afraid of the breast cancer risk', *Climacteric,* 25(4) pp.362-68. doi: 10.1080/13697137.2022.2035711

72. Rossouw, J. E. et al. (2022), 'Risks and benefits of estrogen plus progestin in healthy postmenopausal women: principal results From the Women's Health Initiative randomized controlled trial', *JAMA,* 288 (3), pp. 321–33. doi:10.1001/jama.288.3.321

73. Mueck, A. O., Seeger, H. (2015), 'Estrogen as a new option for prevention and treatment of breast cancer – does this need a "time gap"?', *Climacteric,* 18 (4), pp. 444–7. doi: 10.3109/13697137.2015.1041904

74. Craig Jordan, V. (2015), 'The new biology of estrogen-induced apoptosis applied to treat and prevent breast cancer', *Endocrine-related Cancer,* 22 (1): R1-31. doi:10.1530/ERC-14-0448

75. Glaser, R., Dimitrakakis, C. (2013), 'Testosterone therapy in women: myths and misconceptions', *Maturitas*, 74 (3), pp. 230–4. doi: 10.1016/j.maturitas.2013.01.003

76. NICE (2015), 'Menopause: diagnosis and management', https://www.nice.org.uk/guidance/ng23

77. Glaser, R., Dimitrakakis, C. (2013), 'Testosterone therapy in women: myths and misconceptions', *Maturitas*, 74 (3), pp. 230–4. doi: 10.1016/j.maturitas.2013.01.003

78. Uloko, M., Rahman, F., Puri, L. I., Rubin, R. S. (2022), 'The clinical management of testosterone replacement therapy in postmenopausal women with hypoactive sexual desire disorder: a review', *International Journal of Impotence Research*, doi: 10.1038/s41443-022-00613-0

79. Parish, S. J., Hahn, S. R. (2016), 'Hypoactive sexual desire disorder: A review of epidemiology, biopsychology, diagnosis, and treatment', *Sex Medicine Reviews*, 4 (2) pp. 103–20. doi: 10.1016/j.sxmr.2015.11.009

80. *London Evening Standard* (2012) 'Jane Fonda's fountain of youth is . . . testosterone', https://www.standard.co.uk/news/celebritynews/jane-fonda-s-fountain-of-youth-is-testosterone-7924349.html

81. Nappi, R. E., Palacios, S., Panay, N., Particco, M., Krychman, M. L. (2016), 'Vulvar and vaginal atrophy in four European countries: evidence from the European REVIVE Survey', *Climacteric*, 19 (2) pp. 188–97. doi: 10.3109/13697137.2015.1107039

82. Kingsberg, S. A., Krychman, M., Graham, S., Bernick, B., Mirkin, S. (2017), 'The women's EMPOWER survey: identifying women's perceptions on vulvar and vaginal atrophy and its treatment', *Journal of Sexual Medicine*, 4(3), pp. 413–24. doi: 10.1016/j.jsxm.2017.01.010.

83. The NAMS 2020 GSM Position Statement Editorial Panel (2020), 'The 2020 genitourinary syndrome of menopause position statement of The North American Menopause Society', *Menopause*, 27 (9) pp. 976–92. doi: 10.1097/GME.0000000000001609

84. Portman, D. J., Goldstein, S. R., Kagan, R. (2019), 'Treatment of moderate to severe dyspareunia with intravaginal prasterone therapy: a review', *Climacteric*, 22 (1), pp. 65–72. doi: 10.1080/13697137.2018.1535583

85. Medicines and Healthcare products Regulatory Agency (2022), 'Easier access to locally-applied HRT to treat postmenopausal vaginal symptoms in landmark MHRA reclassification', https://www.gov.uk/government/news/easier-access-to-locally-applied-hrt-to-treat-postmenopausal-vaginal-symptoms-in-landmark-mhra-reclassification

Chapter 5

86. Lejri, I., Grimm, A., Eckert, A. (2018), 'Mitochondria, estrogen and female brain aging', *Frontiers in Aging Neuroscience*, doi: 10.3389/fnagi.2018.00124

87. Bustamante-Barrientos, F. A., Méndez-Ruette, M., Ortloff, A., Luz-Crawford, P., Rivera, F. J., Figueroa, C. D., Molina, L., Bátiz, L. F. (2021), 'The impact of estrogen and estrogen-like molecules in neurogenesis and neurodegeneration: beneficial or harmful?', *Frontiers in Cellular Neurophysiology*, doi: 10.3389/fncel.2021.636176

88. Herson, M., Kulkarni, J. (2022), 'Hormonal agents for the treatment of depression associated with the menopause', *Drugs Aging*, 39 (8), pp. 607–18. doi: 10.1007/s40266-022-00962-x

89. Mirkin, S. (2018), 'Evidence on the use of progesterone in menopausal hormone therapy', *Climacteric*, 21 (4), pp. 346–54. doi: 10.1080/13697137.2018.1455657

90. Glaser, R., Dimitrakakis, C. (2013), 'Testosterone therapy in women: myths and misconceptions', *Maturitas*, 74 (3), pp. 230–4. doi:10.1016/j.maturitas.2013.01.003

91. Studd, J., Nappi, R. E. (2012), 'Reproductive depression', *Gynecological Endocrinology*, vol. 28 suppl. 1, pp. 42–5. doi:10.3109/09513590.2012.651932

92. Freeman, E. W. (2010), 'Associations of depression with the transition to menopause', *Menopause*, 17(4) pp. 823–7. doi:10.1097/gme.0b013e3181db9f8b

93. Herson, M., Kulkarni, J. (2022), 'Hormonal Agents for the Treatment of Depression Associated with the Menopause', *Drugs Aging*, 39 (8) pp. 607–18. doi: 10.1007/s40266-022-00962-x

94. Panay, N., Studd, J. (1997), 'Progestogen intolerance and compliance with hormone replacement therapy in menopausal women', *Human Reproduction Update*, 3(2) pp. 159–71. doi: 10.1093/humupd/3.2.159

95. Ruan, X., Mueck, A. O. (2014), 'Systemic progesterone therapy–oral, vaginal, injections and even transdermal?' *Maturitas*, 79(3), pp. 248–55. doi: 10.1016/j.maturitas.2014.07.009

96. Hardy, C., Griffiths, A., Norton, S., Hunter, M. S. (2018), 'Self-help cognitive behavior therapy for working women with problematic hot flushes and night sweats (MENOS@Work): a multicenter randomized controlled trial', *Menopause*, 25 (5), pp. 508–19. doi: 10.1097/GME.0000000000001048

97. Nowacka-Chmielewska, M., Grabowska, K., Grabowski, M., Meybohm, P.,

Burek, M., Małecki, A. (2022), 'Running from stress: neurobiological mechanisms of exercise-induced stress resilience', *International Journal of Molecular Sciences*, 23(21):13348. doi: 10.3390/ijms232113348

98. Sood, R., Kuhle, C. L., Kapoor, E., Thielen, J. M., Frohmader, K. S., Mara, K. C., Faubion, S. S. (2019), 'Association of mindfulness and stress with menopausal symptoms in midlife women', *Climacteric*, 22 (4), pp. 377–82. doi: 10.1080/13697137.2018.1551344.

99. Ibid.

100. Carmody, J. F., Crawford, S., Salmoirago-Blotcher, E., Leung, K., Churchill, L., Olendzki N. (2011), 'Mindfulness training for coping with hot flashes: results of a randomized trial', *Menopause*, 18 (6), pp. 611–20. doi:10.1097/gme.0b013e318204a05c

101. Leonhardt, M. (2019), 'Low mood and depressive symptoms during perimenopause – Should General Practitioners prescribe hormone replacement therapy or antidepressants as the first-line treatment?', *Post Reproductive Health*, 25 (3) pp. 124–30. doi:10.1177/2053369119847867

102. Westlund, T. L., Parry, B. L. (2003), 'Does estrogen enhance the anti-depressant effects of fluoxetine?', *Journal of Affective Disorders*, 77 (1) pp. 87–92. doi: 10.1016/s0165-0327(02)00357-9. PMID: 14550939

103. Soares, C. N., Almeida, O. P., Joffe, H., Cohen, L. S. (2001), 'Efficacy of estradiol for the treatment of depressive disorders in perimenopausal women: a double-blind, randomized, placebo-controlled trial', *Archives of General Psychiatry*, 58 (6), pp. 529–34. doi: 10.1001/archpsyc.58.6.529. PMID: 11386980

104. Ibid.

105. Riecher-Rössler, A. (2017), 'Oestrogens, prolactin, hypothalamic-pitu-itary-gonadal axis, and schizophrenic psychoses', *Lancet Psychiatry*, 4 (1), pp. 63–72. doi:10.1016/S2215-0366(16)30379-0

106. Moura, C. et al. (2014) 'Antidepressant use and 10-year incident fracture risk: the population-based Canadian Multicentre Osteoporosis Study (CaMoS)', *Osteoporos Int*, 25 (5) pp. 1473–81, doi: 10.1007/s00198-014-2649-x

107. Dorani, F., Bijlenga, D., Beekman, A. T. F., van Someren, E. J. W., Kooij, J. J. S. (2021), 'Prevalence of hormone-related mood disorder symptoms in women with ADHD', *Journal of Psychiatric Research*, 133: pp. 10–15. doi: 10.1016/j.jpsychires.2020.12.005

108. Palagini, L. et al. (2013), 'REM sleep dysregulation in depression: state of the art', *Sleep Medicine Reviews*, 17 (5) pp. 377–90. doi:10.1016/j.smrv.2012.11.001

Chapter 6

109. National Hair and Beauty Federation (2021), 'NHBF industry research and statistics 2021', www.nhbf.co.uk/about-the-nhbf/what-we-do/industry-research

110. Leitch, C. et al. (2011), 'Women's perceptions of the effects of menopause and hormone replacement therapy on skin', *Menopause International*, 17 (1), pp. 11–13. doi:10.1258/mi.2011.011002

111. Thornton, M. J. (2013), 'Estrogens and aging skin', *Dermato-endocrinology*, 5 (2), pp. 264–70. doi:10.4161/derm.23872

112. Donley, G. M., Liu, W. T., Pfeiffer, R. M., McDonald, E. C., Peters, K. O., Tucker, M. A., Cahoon, E. K. (2019), 'Reproductive factors, exogenous hormone use and incidence of melanoma among women in the United States', *British Journal of Cancer*, 120 (7), pp. 754–60. doi: 10.1038/s41416-019-0411-z

113. Callens, A. et al. (1996), 'Does hormonal skin aging exist? A study of the influence of different hormone therapy regimens on the skin of postmenopausal women using non-invasive measurement techniques', *Dermatology*, 193 (4), pp. 289–94. doi:10.1159/000246272

114. Windhager, S., Mitteroecker, P., Rupić, I., Lauc, T., Polašek, O., Schaefer, K. (2019), 'Facial aging trajectories: A common shape pattern in male and female faces is disrupted after menopause', *American Journal of Physical Anthropology*, 169 (4), pp. 678–88. doi:10.1002/ajpa.23878

115. Thornton, M. J. (2013), 'Estrogens and aging skin', *Dermato-endocrinology*, 5 (2), pp. 264–70. doi:10.4161/derm.23872

116. Shapiro, J. (2007), 'Clinical practice. Hair loss in women', *New England Journal of Medicine*, 357 (16), pp. 1620–30 doi:10.1056/NEJMcp072110

117. Goluch-Koniuszy, Z. S. (2016), 'Nutrition of women with hair loss problem during the period of menopause', *Przeglad Menopauzalny*, 15 (1), pp. 56–61. doi:10.5114/pm.2016.58776

Chapter 7

118. The Daisy Network, 'What is POI?', https://www.daisynetwork.org/about-poi/what-is-poi

119. Baber, R. J., Panay, N., Fenton, A. (2016), 'IMS Writing Group. 2016 IMS Recommendations on women's midlife health and menopause hormone therapy', *Climacteric*, 19 (2) pp. 109–50. doi: 10.3109/13697137.2015.1129166

120. Moorman, P. G., Myers, E. R., Schildkraut, J. M., Iversen, E. S., Wang, F., Warren, N. (2011), 'Effect of hysterectomy with ovarian preservation on ovarian function', *Obstetrics and Gynecology*, 118 (6) pp. 1271–9. doi: 10.1097/AOG.0b013e318236fd12

121. Sullivan, S. D., Sarrel, P. M., Nelson, L. M. (2016), 'Hormone replacement therapy in young women with primary ovarian insufficiency and early menopause', *Fertility and Sterility*, 106 (7) pp. 1588–99. doi: 10.1016/j.fertnstert.2016.09.046

122. Sarrel, P. M., Sullivan, S. D., Nelson, L. M. (2016), 'Hormone replacement therapy in young women with surgical primary ovarian insufficiency', *Fertility and Sterility*, 106(7) pp. 1580–7. doi: 10.1016/j.fertnstert.2016.09.018

123. Rocca, W. A. et al. (2016), 'Accelerated Accumulation of Multimorbidity After Bilateral Oophorectomy: A Population-Based Cohort Study', *Mayo Clinic Proceedings*, 91 (11), pp. 1577–89. doi:10.1016/j.mayocp.2016.08.002

Chapter 8

124. Ferlay, J. et al. (2018), 'Estimating the global cancer incidence and mortality in 2018: GLOBOCAN sources and methods', *International Journal of Cancer*, 144 (8), pp. 1941–53. doi:10.1002/ijc.31937

125. National Institutes of Health: National Cancer Institute Surveillance, Epidemiology, and End Results Program (2022), 'Cancer Stat Facts: Female Breast Cancer', https://seer.cancer.gov/statfacts/html/breast.html

126. Bell, R. J. (2019), 'Ringing the bell and then falling off a cliff ... life after cancer', *Climacteric*, 22 (6) pp. 533–4. doi: 10.1080/13697137.2019.1576456. PMID: 31612747

127. Bounous, V. et al (2020), 'Cognition and early menopause in breast cancer patients: an update', *Gynecological and Reproductive Endocrinology and Metabolism*, 1(1) pp. 23–28

128. Jackson, S. E. et al. (2016), 'Sexuality after a cancer diagnosis: a population-based study', *Cancer*, 122 (24), pp. 3883–91. doi:10.1002/cncr.30263

129. Ibid.

130. Langer, R. D. (2021), 'The role of medications in successful aging', *Climacteric*, 24 (5) pp. 505–12. doi: 10.1080/13697137.2021.1911991

131. Macmillan Cancer Support (2022), 'Tiredness (fatigue)', https://www.macmillan.org.uk/cancer-information-and-support/impacts-of-cancer/tiredness

132. Kings College Hospital NHS Foundation Trust (2021) 'Sleep Hygiene', https: //www.kch.nhs.uk/Doc/pl%20-%20947.1%20-%20sleep%20hygiene.pdf

133. Pitman, A., Suleman, S., Hyde, N., Hodgkiss, A. (2018), 'Depression and anxiety in patients with cancer', *BMJ*, doi: 10.1136/bmj.k1415. PMID: 29695476

134. Papadimitriou, N. et al. (2020), 'Physical activity and risks of breast and colorectal cancer: a Mendelian randomisation analysis', *Nature Communications*, 11 (1) 597, doi:10.1038/s41467-020-14389-8

135. Edwards, D., Panay, N. (2016), 'Treating vulvovaginal atrophy/genitourinary syndrome of menopause: how important is vaginal lubricant and moisturizer composition?' *Climacteric*, 19(2) pp. 151–61. doi: 10.3109/13697137.2015.1124259

136. Hirschberg, A. L. et al. (2021), 'Topical estrogens and non-hormonal preparations for postmenopausal vulvovaginal atrophy: An EMAS clinical guide', *Maturitas*, 148, pp. 55–61. doi:10.1016/j.maturitas.2021.04.005

137. Laing, A. J., Newson, L., Simon, J. A. (2022), 'Individual benefits and risks of intravaginal estrogen and systemic testosterone in the management of women in the menopause, with a discussion of any associated risks for cancer development', *Cancer*, 28 (3), pp. 196–203. doi: 10.1097/PPO.0000000000000598. PMID: 35594467

138. Pinkerton, J. V., Santen, R. J. (2019), 'Managing vasomotor symptoms in women after cancer', *Climacteric*, 22(6) pp. 544–52. doi: 10.1080/13697137.2019.1600501

139. Hunter, M. S. (2021), 'Cognitive behavioral therapy for menopausal symptoms', *Climacteric*, 24 (1), pp. 51–6. doi: 10.1080/13697137.2020

140. Carmona, N. E., Millett, G. E., Green, S. M., Carney, C. E. (2022), 'Cognitive-behavioral, behavioral and mindfulness-based therapies for insomnia in menopause', *Behavioral Sleep Medicine*, Aug 9, pp. 1–12. doi: 10.1080/15402002.2022.2109640

141. Szabo, R. A., Marino, J. L., Hickey, M. (2019), 'Managing menopausal symptoms after cancer', *Climacteric*, 22 (6), pp. 572–8. doi: 10.1080/13697137.2019.1646718. Epub 2019 Aug 21. PMID: 31433675

142. Azizi, M., Khani, S., Kamali, M., Elyasi, F. (2022), 'The efficacy and safety of selective serotonin reuptake inhibitors and serotonin-norepinephrine reuptake inhibitors in the treatment of menopausal hot flashes: a systematic review of clinical trials', *Iran Journal of Medical Sciences*, 47(3), pp. 173–93. doi: 10.30476/ijms.2020.87687.1817

143. Juurlink, D. (2016), 'Revisiting the drug interaction between tamoxifen and SSRI antidepressants', *BMJ*. doi:10.1136/bmj.i5309

144. Ferguson, J. M. (2001), 'SSRI antidepressant medications: adverse effects and tolerability', *Primary care companion to the Journal of Clinical Psychiatry*, 3 (1), pp. 22–7. doi:10.4088/pcc.v03n0105

145. Pandya, K. J., Morrow, G. R., Roscoe, J. A. et al. (2005), 'Gabapentin for hot flashes in 420 women with breast cancer: a randomised double-blind placebo-controlled trial', *Lancet*. 366 (9488) pp. 818–24. doi:10.1016/S0140-6736(05)67215-7

146. British Menopause Society (2022), 'Prescribable alternatives to HRT' https://thebms.org.uk/wp-content/uploads/2022/06/02-BMS-TfC-Prescribable-alternatives-to-HRT-03A-JUNE2022.pdf

147. Rocca, W. A. et al. (2016), 'Accelerated accumulation of multimorbidity after bilateral oophorectomy: a population-based cohort study', *Mayo Clinic Proceedings*, 91 (11) pp. 1577–89. doi:10.1016/j.mayocp.2016.08.002

148. Ossewaarde, M. E. et al. (2005), 'Age at menopause, cause-specific mortality and total life expectancy', *Epidemiology*, 16 (4), pp. 556–62. doi:10.1097/01.ede.0000165392.35273.d4

149. Langer, R. D. (2021), 'The role of medications in successful aging', *Climacteric*, 24 (5) pp. 505–12. doi: 10.1080/13697137.2021.1911991

150. The Eve Appeal, 'Gynaecological cancers', https://eveappeal.org.uk/gynaecological-cancers/#:~:text=Each%20year%20in%20the%20UK,day%20from%20their%20gynaecological%20cancer

151. MacLennan, A. H. (2011), 'HRT in difficult circumstances: are there any absolute contraindications?', *Climacteric*, 14(4) pp. 409–17, doi: 10.3109/13697137.2010.543496

152. Mascarenhas, C. et al (2006), 'Use of hormone replacement therapy before and after ovarian cancer diagnosis and ovarian cancer survival', *International Journal of Cancer*, 119 (12), pp. 2907–15. doi:10.1002/ijc.22218

153. Eeles, R. A, et al. (2015), 'Adjuvant hormone therapy may improve survival in epithelial ovarian cancer: results of the AHT randomized trial', *Journal of Clinical Oncology*, 33 (35) pp. 4138–44. doi: 10.1200/JCO.2015.60.9719

154. Pergialiotis, V. et al. (2016), 'Hormone therapy for ovarian cancer survivors: systematic review and meta-analysis', *Menopause*, 23 (3), pp. 335–42. doi: 10.1097/GME.0000000000000508

155. Deli, T., Orosz, M., Jakab, A. (2020), 'Hormone replacement therapy in cancer survivors – review of the literature', *Pathology Oncology Research*, 26 (1), pp. 63–78. doi: 10.1007/s12253-018-00569-x. Epub 2019 Jan 8. PMID: 30617760; PMCID: PMC7109141

156 Singh P., Oehler, M. K. (2010), 'Hormone replacement after gynaecological cancer', *Maturitas*, 65 (3), pp. 190–7. doi:10.1016/j.maturitas.2009.11.017

157. Hinds, L., Price, J. (2010), 'Menopause, hormone replacement and gynaecological cancers', *Menopause International*, 16 (2), pp. 89–93. doi: 10.1258/mi.2010.010018

158. Deli T., Orosz, M., Jakab, A. (2020), 'Hormone replacement therapy in cancer survivors – review of the literature', *Pathology Oncology Research*, 26 (1), pp. 63–78. doi: 10.1007/s12253-018-00569-x. Epub 2019 Jan 8. PMID: 30617760; PMCID: PMC7109141

159. Hinds, L., Price J. (2010), 'Menopause, hormone replacement and gynae-cological cancers', *Menopause International*, 16 (2), pp. 89–93. doi: 10.1258/mi.2010.010018

160. Falk, S. J., Dizon, D. S. (2020), 'Sexual Health Issues in Cancer Survivors. *Seminars in Oncology Nursing*, Feb;36(1):150981. doi: 10.1016/j.soncn.2019.150981. Epub 2020 Jan 24. PMID: 31983486

161. National Institute for Health and Care Excellence (2015), 'Menopause: diagnosis and management', https://www.nice.org.uk/guidance/ng23

162. Raglan, G. B., Schulkin, J., Micks, E. (2020), 'Depression during peri-menopause: the role of the obstetrician-gynecologist', *Archives of Women's Mental Health*, 23 (1) pp. 1–10. doi: 10.1007/s00737-019-0950-6. Epub 2019 Feb 13. PMID: 30758732

163. Zhao, F. Y., Fu, Q. Q., Spencer, S. J. et al. (2021), 'Acupuncture: a promis-ing approach for comorbid depression and insomnia in perimenopause', *Nature and Science of Sleep*, 13, pp. 1823–63. doi:10.2147/NSS.S332474

164. National Institute for Health and Care Excellence (2018), 'Early and locally advanced breast cancer: diagnosis and management', www.nice.org.uk/guidance/ng101

165. Berliere, M., Duhoux, F. P., Dalenc, F. et al. (2013), 'Tamoxifen and ovarian function', *PLoS One*, 8 (6): e66616. doi:10.1371/journal.pone.0066616

166. National Institute for Health and Care Excellence (2018), 'Early and locally advanced breast cancer: diagnosis and management', www.nice.org.uk/guidance/ng101

167. Bluming, A., (2022), 'Hormone replacement therapy after breast cancer: it is time', *Cancer Journal*, 28 (3), pp. 183–90, doi: 10.1097/PPO.0000000000000595

168. Holmberg, L., Anderson, H. (2004), 'HABITS steering and data monitor-ing committees. HABITS (hormonal replacement therapy after breast cancer--is it safe?), a randomised comparison: trial stopped', *Lancet*, 7;363(9407), pp. 453–5. doi: 10.1016/S0140-6736(04)15493-7

169. (2016), 'ACOG Committee Opinion No. 659: The use of vaginal estrogen in women with a history of estrogen-dependent breast cancer', *Obstetrics and Gynecology*, 127 (3) e93–6. doi:10.1097/AOG.0000000000001351

170. All-Party Parliamentary Group on Menopause (2022), 'Inquiry to assess the impacts of menopause and the case for policy reform: concluding report', https://menopause-appg.co.uk/wp-content/uploads/2022/10/APPG-Menopause-Inquiry-Concluding-Report-12.10.22-1.pdF

171. Cancer Research UK (2020), 'Family history of breast cancer and inherited genes', https://www.cancerresearchuk.org/about-cancer/breast-cancer/risks-causes/family-history-and-inherited-genes#:~:text=This%20is%20called%20a%20family,under%20the%20age%20of%2050

172. Kotsopoulos, J. et al. (2018), 'Hormone replacement therapy after oophorectomy and breast cancer risk among BRCA1 mutation carriers', *JAMA Oncology*, 4 (8) pp. 1059–65. doi:10.1001/jamaoncol.2018.0211

173. Vermeulen, R. F. M. et al. (2019), 'Safety of hormone replacement therapy following risk-reducing salpingo-oophorectomy: systematic review of literature and guidelines', *Climacteric*, pp. 352–60. doi:10.1080/13697137.2019.1582622

174. General Medical Council (2020), 'Decision Making and Consent', https://www.gmc-uk.org/ethical-guidance/ethical-guidance-for-doctors/decision-making-and-consent

175. National Institute for Health and Care Excellence (2021), 'Shared Decision Making', https://www.nice.org.uk/guidance/ng197

Chapter 9

176. Harlow, S. D. et al. (2022), 'Disparities in reproductive aging and midlife health between black and white women: The Study of Women's Health Across the Nation (SWAN)', *Women's Midlife Health*. doi:10.1186/s40695-022-00073-y

177. American Heart Association (2021), 'Early menopause linked to higher risk of future coronary heart disease', https://newsroom.heart.org/news/early-menopause-linked-to-higher-risk-of-future-coronary-heart-disease?preview=f0f8

178. Gold, E. B. (2011), 'The timing of the age at which natural menopause occurs', *Obstetrics and Gynecology*, 38 (3) pp. 425–40. doi: 10.1016/j.ogc.2011.05.002

179. Im, E. O. et al. (2010), 'Menopausal symptoms among four major ethnic groups in the United States', *Western Journal of Nursing Research*, 32 (4), pp. 540–65. doi:10.1177/0193945909354343

180. Chen, M. N., Lin, C. C., Liu, C. F. (2015), 'Efficacy of phytoestrogens for menopausal symptoms: a meta-analysis and systematic review', *Climacteric*, 18(2), pp.260–9. doi.org/10.3109/13697137.2014.966241

181. Hu, D., Yu, D. (2010), 'Epidemiology of cardiovascular disease in Asian women', *Nutrition, Metabolism, and Cardiovascular Diabetes*, 20(6), pp. 394–404. doi.org/10.1016/j.numecd.2010.02.016

182. Diversity.org.uk, 'Diversity in the UK', https://diversityuk.org/diversity-in-the-uk

183. The Fawcett Society (2022), 'Menopause and the Workplace', www.fawcettsociety.org.uk/menopauseandtheworkplace

184. Diversity.org.uk, 'Diversity in the UK', https://diversityuk.org/diversity-in-the-uk

185. Ipsos (2022), 'Global views on menopause', https://www.ipsos.com/sites/default/files/ct/news/documents/2022-10/Ipsos-Global%20Views%20on%20Menopause.pdf

186. Stonewall (2018), 'LGBT in Britain: Health Report', www.stonewall.org.uk/system/files/lgbt_in_britain_health.pdf

187. Ibid.

188. Solomon, D., Sabin, C. A., Burns, F., Gilson, R., Allan, S., de Ruiter, A., Dhairyawan, R., Fox, J., Gilleece, Y., Jones, R., Post, F., Reeves, I., Ross, J., Ustianowski, A., Shepherd, J., Tariq, S. (2021), 'The association between severe menopausal symptoms and engagement with HIV care and treatment in women living with HIV', *AIDS Care*, 33(1), pp. 101–8. doi: 10.1080/09540121.2020.1748559

189. Unicef (2016), 'Female genital mutilation/cutting: a global concern', https://data.unicef.org/resources/female-genital-mutilationcutting-global-concern

190. Office for Health Improvement and Disparities (2021), 'Female genital mutilation (FGM): migrant health guide', www.gov.uk/guidance/female-genital-mutilation-fgm-migrant-health-guide

191. Farage, M. A., Miller, K. W., Tzeghai, G. E., Azuka, C. E., Sobel, J. D., Ledger, W. J. (2015), 'Female genital cutting: confronting cultural challenges and health complications across the lifespan', *Womens Health*, 11 (1), pp. 79–94. doi: 10.2217/whe.14.63. PMID: 25581057

192. Allsworth, J. E., Zierler, S., Lapane, K. L., Krieger, N., Hogan, J. W., Harlow, B. L. (2004), 'Longitudinal study of the inception of perimenopause in relation to lifetime history of sexual or physical violence', *Journal of Epidemiology and Community Health*, 58 (11) pp. 938–43. doi: 10.1136/jech.2003.017160

193. Gipson, C. D., Bimonte-Nelson, H. A. (2021), 'Interactions between reproductive transitions during aging and addiction: promoting translational crosstalk between different fields of research', *Behavioural Pharmacology*, 32(2&3), pp. 112–22. doi: 10.1097/FBP.0000000000000591

Chapter 10

194. Nuffield Health (2022), 'The Nuffield Health Healthier Nation Index', https://www.nuffieldhealth.com/healthiernation#key-insights
195. Armstrong, M. E. G. et al. (2015), 'Frequent physical activity may not reduce vascular disease risk as much as moderate activity: large prospective study of women in the United Kingdom', *Circulation*, vol. 131(8), pp. 721–9. doi:10.1161/CIRCULATIONAHA.114.010296
196. Saint-Maurice, P. F. et al. (2020), 'Association of daily step count and step intensity with mortality among US adults', *JAMA*, 323 (12), pp. 1151–60. doi:10.1001/jama.2020.1382
197. Akyuz, A. (2020), 'Exercise and coronary heart disease', *Advances in Experimental Medicine and Biology*, 1228, pp. 169–79. doi:10.1007/978-981-15-1792-1_11
198. Alzheimer's UK, 'Physical exercise and dementia', https://www.alzheimers.org.uk/about-dementia/risk-factors-and-prevention/physical-exercise
199. Benedetti, M. G. et al (2018), 'The effectiveness of physical exercise on bone density in osteoporotic patients', *BioMed Research International*, doi.org/10.1155/2018/4840531
200. Pinheiro, M. B., Oliveira, J., Bauman, A. et al. (2020), 'Evidence on physical activity and osteoporosis prevention for people aged 65+ years: a systematic review to inform the WHO guidelines on physical activity and sedentary behaviour', *International Journal of Behavioral Nutrition and Physical Activity*, doi.org/10.1186/s12966-020-01040-4
201. Dolezal, B. A. et al. (2017), 'Interrelationship between sleep and exercise: a systematic review', *Advances in Preventive Medicine*, doi:10.1155/2017/1364387
202. Kelley, G. A., Kelley, K. (2017), 'Exercise and sleep: a systematic review of previous meta-analyses', *Journal of Evidence-based Medicine*, 10 (1), pp. 26–36. doi:10.1111/jebm.12236
203. Department of Health and Social Care and Office for Health Improvement and Disparities (2022), 'Physical activity guidelines', www.gov.uk/government/collections/physical-activity-guidelines

204. Jorge, M. P. et al. (2016), 'Hatha Yoga practice decreases menopause symptoms and improves quality of life: A randomized controlled trial', *Complementary Therapies in Medicine*, 26, pp. 128–35. doi:10.1016/j.ctim.2016.03.014

205. Cramer, H. et al. (2018), 'Yoga for menopausal symptoms – A systematic review and meta-analysis', *Maturitas*, 109, pp. 13–25. doi:10.1016/j.maturitas.2017.12.005

206. Gov.uk (2022), 'Physical activity', www.ethnicity-facts-figures.service.gov.uk/health/diet-and-exercise/physical-activity/latest

207. Department for Work and Pensions (2021), 'Family Resources Survey', https://www.gov.uk/government/collections/family-resources-survey--2

Chapter 11

208. De Cabo, R., Mattson, M. P. (2019), 'Effects of intermittent fasting on health, aging, and disease', *New England Journal of Medicine*, 381(26), pp. 2541–51, doi.org/10.1056/NEJMra1905136

209. Public Health England (2016), 'Government Dietary Recommendations', https://assets.publishing.service.gov.uk/government/uploads/system/uploads/attachment_data/file/618167/government_dietary_recommendations.pdf

210. University of Edinburgh, 'Calcium calculator', https://webapps.igmm.ed.ac.uk/world/research/rheumatological/calcium-calculator/

211. Kaviani, M., Nikooyeh, B., Etesam, F., Behnagh, S. J., Kangarani, H. M., Arefi, M., Yaghmaei, P., Neyestani, T. R. (2022), 'Effects of vitamin D supplementation on depression and some selected pro-inflammatory biomarkers: a double-blind randomized clinical trial', *BMC Psychiatry*, 22(1): 694.doi: 10.1186/s12888-022-04305-3

212. Yousefi, R. E., Djalali, M., Koohdani, F., Saboor-Yaraghi, A. A., Eshraghian, M.R., Javanbakht, M. H., Saboori, S., Zarei, M., Hosseinzadeh-Attar, M. J. (2014), 'The effects of vitamin D supplementation on glucose control and insulin resistance in patients with diabetes type 2: a randomized clinical trial study', *Iranian Journal of Public Health*, 43(12) pp. 1651–6

213. Department of Health and Social Care (2021), 'Vitamin D and clinically extremely vulnerable (CEV) guidance', www.gov.uk/government/publications/vitamin-d-for-vulnerable-groups/vitamin-d-and-clinically-extremely-vulnerable-cev-guidance#:~:text=Advice%20on%20the%20recommended%20dose&text=10%20micrograms%20of%20

vitamin%20D%20is%20a%20safe%20level%20of,per%20day%20is%20considered%20safe

214. Wang, H., Chen, W., Li, D., Yin, X., Zhang, X., Olsen, N., Zheng, S. G. (2017), 'Vitamin D and chronic diseases', *Aging and Disease*, 8 (3) pp. 346–53. doi: 10.14336/AD.2016.1021

215. Yang, Q., Jian, J., Katz, S., Abramson, S. B., Huang, X. (2012), '17β-Estradiol inhibits iron hormone hepcidin through an estrogen responsive element half-site', *Endocrinology*, 153(7) pp. 3170–8. doi: 10.1210/en.2011-2045

216. National Institute for Health and Care Excellence (2021), 'Anaemia – iron deficiency: How common is it?', https://cks.nice.org.uk/topics/anaemia-iron-deficiency/background-information/prevalence/

217. Cook, J. D., Skikne, B. S., Baynes, R. D. (1994), 'Iron deficiency: the global perspective', *Advances in Experimental Medicine and Biology*, 356, pp. 219–28, doi.org/10.1007/978-1-4615-2554-7_24

218. Public Health England (2016), 'Government Dietary Recommendations', https://assets.publishing.service.gov.uk/government/uploads/system/uploads/attachment_data/file/618167/government_dietary_recommen-dations.pdf

219. NHS.uk (2022), 'How to get more fibre into your diet', https://www.nhs.uk/live-well/eat-well/digestive-health/how-to-get-more-fibre-into-your-diet/#:~:text=Government%20guidelines%20say%20our%20dietary,ways%20of%20increasing%20our%20intake.

220. Public Health England (2016), 'Government Dietary Recommendations', https://assets.publishing.service.gov.uk/government/uploads/system/uploads/attachment_data/file/618167/government_dietary_recommen-dations.pdf

221. Harvard School of Public Health, 'Nutrition source: avocadoes', www.hsph.harvard.edu/nutritionsource/avocados/#:~:text=A%20whole%20medium%20avocado%20contains,levels%2C%20avoca-dos%20contain%20no%20cholesterol

222. Abildgaard, J., Ploug, T., Al-Saoudi, E., Wagner, T., Thomsen, C., Ewertsen, C., Bzorek, M., Pedersen, B. K., Pedersen, A. T., Lindegaard, B. (2021), 'Changes in abdominal subcutaneous adipose tissue phenotype following menopause is associated with increased visceral fat mass', *Scientific Reports*, 11(1):14750. doi: 10.1038/s41598-021-94189-2

223. Zhu, D., Chung, H. F., Dobson, A.J., Pandeya, N., Brunner, E. J., Kuh, D., Greenwood, D. C., Hardy, R., Cade, J. E., Giles, G. G., Bruinsma, F., Demakakos, P., Simonsen, M. K., Sandin, S., Weiderpass, E., Mishra, G. D.

(2020), 'Type of menopause, age of menopause and variations in the risk of incident cardiovascular disease: pooled analysis of individual data from 10 international studies', *Human Reproduction*, 35(8), pp. 1933–43. doi: 10.1093/humrep/deaa124

224. Christakis, M. K., Hasan, H., de Souza, L. R., Shirreff, L. (2020), 'The effect of menopause on metabolic syndrome: cross-sectional results from the Canadian Longitudinal Study on Aging', *Menopause*, 27 (9) pp. 999–1009. doi: 10.1097/GME.0000000000001575

225. Gruzdeva, O., Borodkina, D., Uchasova, E., Dyleva, Y., Barbarash, O. (2018), 'Localization of fat depots and cardiovascular risk', *Lipids in Health and Disease*, 17(1):218. doi: 10.1186/s12944-018-0856-8

226. Dalal, P. K., Agarwal, M. (2015), 'Postmenopausal syndrome', *Indian Journal of Psychiatry*, 57(Suppl. 2):S222–32. doi: 10.4103/0019 -5545.161483

227. Dumas, J. A., Makarewicz, J. A., Bunn, J., Nickerson, J., McGee, E. (2018), 'Dopamine-dependent cognitive processes after menopause: the relationship between COMT genotype, estradiol, and working memory', *Neurobiology of Aging*, 72:53-61. doi: 10.1016/j.neurobiolaging. 2018.08.009

228. Bermingham, K. M., Linenberg, I., Hall, W. L., Kadé, K., Franks, P. W., Davies, R., Wolf, J., Hadjigeorgiou, G., Asnicar, F., Segata, N., Manson, J. E., Newson, L. R., Delahanty, L. M., Ordovas, J. M., Chan, A. T., Spector, T. D., Valdes, A. M., Berry, S. E. (2022), 'Menopause is associated with postprandial metabolism, metabolic health and lifestyle: The ZOE PREDICT study', *EBioMedicine*, 85:104303. doi: 10.1016/j.ebiom.2022.104303

229. Park, S. et al. (2017), 'Lactobacillus plantarum HAC01 regulates gut microbiota and adipose tissue accumulation in a diet-induced obesity murine model', *Applied Microbiology and Biotechnology*, 101 (4), pp. 1605–14. doi:10.1007/s00253-016-7953-2

230. Nagy-Szakal, D. et al. (2017), 'Fecal metagenomic profiles in subgroups of patients with myalgic encephalomyelitis/chronic fatigue syndrome', *Microbiome*, 5 (1) doi:10.1186/s40168-017-0261-y

Chapter 12

231. Women and Equalities Committee (2022), 'Menopause and the workplace', https://publications.parliament.uk/pa/cm5803/cmselect/cmwomeq/91/report.html

232. Newson, L., Lewis, R. (2021), 'Impact of Perimenopause and Menopause on

Work', https://balance-website-prod.s3-eu-west-1.amazonaws.com/uploads/2021/10/Menopause-and-work-poster-RCGP.pdf

233. Newson, L., Chatwin, L., Lews, R., Reisel, D. (2022), 'Impact of meno-pausal symptoms on the working lives of women: a survey of NHS employees in the UK'. Presented at International Menopause Society World Congress on Menopause 2022, www.nhmenopausesociety.org/newson-health-team-to-showcase-new-research-and-insights-at-global-conference

234. Lewis, R., Lalahy, G, Chatwin, L., Reisel, D., Newson, L. (2022), 'Future in our hands: free balance™ app empowers women to become their own advocates'. Presented at International Menopause Society World Congress on Menopause 2022, www.nhmenopausesociety.org/newson-health-team-to-showcase-new-research-and-insights-at-global-conference

235. World Economic Forum (2022), 'Global Gender Gap Report 2022', www.weforum.org/reports/global-gender-gap-report-2022

236. Balance (2022), 'Menopause Cripples the UK economy', www.balance-menopause.com/news/menopause-cripples-the-uk-economy

Conclusion

237. Hillman, S., Shantikumar, S., Ridha, A., Todkill, D., Dale, J. (2020), 'Socioeconomic status and HRT prescribing: a study of practice-level data in England', *British Journal of General Practice*, 70 (700):e772–7. doi: 10.3399/bjgp20X713045

238. Abenhaim, H. A. et al. (2022), 'Menopausal hormone therapy formula-tion and breast cancer risk', *Obstetrics and Gynecology*, 139 (6), pp. 1103–10. doi:10.1097/AOG.0000000000004723

239. Hill, K. (1996), 'The demography of menopause', *Maturitas*, 23(2), pp. 113–27. doi.org/10.1016/0378-5122(95)00968-x

Index

abdominal pain 42–3
acne 164–5, 167–8, 172, 178
actives 172, 173
acupuncture 220
addiction 237, 254
adrenal glands 10, 11, 13
adrenaline 43, 300
ageing 11–12, 97, 170, 173
alcohol 21, 57, 61, 98, 214, 254, 281
Alzheimer's 12, 97, 104, 106, 261
anaemia, iron-deficiency 286–7, 289
antidepressants 137, 147–8, 150–1, 159, 214–15
anxiety 60, 144, 145, 147, 152, 157, 158, 205, 206–7, 283, 300
Arif, Dr Nighat 255
aromatase inhibitors 182, 204, 208, 223
artichoke and chickpea dip 319–20
Aujla, Dr Rupy 321–2
avocados: mint, avocado and bean salad 313–14

Ball, Dr Sarah 227
beans: mint, avocado and bean salad 313–14
beetroot: roasted beetroot and cauliflower salad 311–12

berries: mood-boosting berry smoothie 309
pink oats with kefir 309–10
Black women, menopause and 238, 240, 246–7
bladders, overactive 65–6
bleeding 43–4, 111, 206
bloating 42–3, 55, 111, 278, 298
blood clots 119–20
blood pressure 99–100, 101–2, 104
blood sugar levels 283, 291, 292
blood tests 189–90
the blues 24–6, 28, 111
body scans 145
bone health 170
  calcium 10, 98, 281–2, 283
  DEXA scans 190–1
  exercise and 211, 261, 271
  hormones and 11, 13, 98
  osteoporosis 12, 97–8, 116, 191, 192, 197, 210, 216, 217, 281
  vitamin D and 283, 293
  yoga and 264, 271
bowel cancer 103, 217
brain fog 13, 44–5, 94, 96, 105, 123, 205, 207, 333
breast cancer 202–3, 205, 211, 220, 222–32

aromatase inhibitors and
    tamoxifen 208, 222–3
barriers to good menopause care
    225–7
family history of 231–2
HRT and 94, 117–19, 120–1,
    223–5, 231, 232
breastfeeding, HRT and 112–14
breasts 11, 39, 46–7, 111
breath, bad 51–2, 55
breathing difficulties 48, 56
Brown, Claudia 143–7
bruising 169

caffeine 21, 47, 57, 61
calcium 10, 98, 212, 281–2, 283
    calcium-rich Parmesan oatcakes
        318–19
cancer 97, 104, 202–35, 285
    and early menopause 76, 77, 183,
        184–7, 204
    finding support 234–5
    how cancer affects the menopause
        204–9, 210–12
    HRT and 94, 120–1, 215–19,
        233
    menopause treatment options
        212–17, 232–4
    see also individual types of cancer
carbohydrates 292–3
cardiovascular disease 97, 99–101,
    116, 192, 210, 217, 260
cauliflower: roasted beetroot and
    cauliflower salad 311–12
ceramides 163, 166
cervical cancer 221–2
cheese: calcium-rich Parmesan
    oatcakes 318–19
chemical menopause 253

chemotherapy 183, 184, 185, 204,
    206, 228
chickpeas: artichoke and chickpea
    dip 319–20
children, broaching the menopause
    with 83, 86, 87–92, 355–6
cholesterol 100, 283, 298
cleansers 166, 172, 174
cognitive behavioural therapy (CBT)
    141–2, 214
cold therapy 47
collagen 163, 166, 169, 170, 173
comfort in a bowl 316–18
concentration 32, 60, 123
constipation 42–3, 289
contraceptive pill 78, 114, 192, 193
cortisol 43, 55, 60, 300
cultural barriers, breaking down
    241–2
Curtis, Matthew 175–6

Daisy Network 198
death, HRT and 103
dementia 104–6, 116, 192, 210, 216,
    261
depression 97, 113, 116, 152, 205,
    283
    clinical 147, 151, 192, 210, 217
    and HRT 148–50, 159
    perimenopause and menopause-
        related 60, 136, 137, 139–59
    postnatal depression (PND) 26–7,
        139, 152
    sleep and 157–8
    treatment options 140–50
DEXA scans 190–1
diabetes 102–3, 104, 116, 183, 192,
    210, 216, 217, 283, 285, 298
diarrhoea 42–3

diet *see* nutrition and diet
digestion 42–3, 55, 262
dip, artichoke and chickpea 319–20
dizziness 48–9, 54, 56
domestic abuse 253
DUTCH test 191

Earle, Liz 337–9, 352
early menopause 97, 179–201
  cancer and 76, 77, 183, 184–7,
    204, 221–2
  and fertility 194–201
  HRT and 186, 192–4, 196–7, 216
  investigation and diagnosis
    188–91
  long-term health risks of 191–2
  treatment options 192–4
  what causes it 182–4
  what it is 181
eating disorders 254
education, menopause 85–6, 355
eggs 37–8, 39
Ellice-Flint, Emma 305–8
endocrine glands 9–10
endorphins 142, 271
energy levels 96, 123, 290, 307
ethnic minorities 238–47
exercise 47, 211, 214, 257–74
  and better health and wellbeing
    259–62
  as bone protection 261, 271
  building an exercise habit 263,
    272
  cancer recovery and 211–12
  dementia and 106, 261
  heart benefits 260–1, 271
  joint pain and 298, 300
  mental health benefits 142–3, 152,
    270, 271

and sleep 261–2, 264
strength training 270, 271
to boost self-esteem 125–6
eyes, dry 49–50

family menopause discussions 79–92,
  355–6
fatigue 94, 96, 123, 199, 205, 207,
  211, 285, 291, 292, 307, 326
fats 293–5
female genital mutilation (FGM)
  251–2
fertility 194–201, 210
fibre 291–2
fish: mint, avocado and bean salad
  with crispy fish 313–14
  sesame-crusted salmon with ginger
    and mint slaw 314–16
flushing 167
follicle-stimulating hormone (FSH)
  12, 189–90, 253
food diaries 278
formication 167, 178

gabapentin 215
Garley, Dr David 157–9
gastrointestinal symptoms 42–3
genetic influences 76, 77, 80
genitourinary syndrome of the
  menopause (GSM) 71, 229, 251
ghrelin 290, 300–1
Gibbs, Rebecca 195–8
ginger and mint slaw 314–16
gingivitis 51, 52, 53
glycaemic index (GI) 292–3
gonadotropin-releasing hormone
  (GnRH) analogues 20
greens: comfort in a bowl 316–18
gum disease 51–2

gut health 304–20
gynaecological cancers 217–19

hair 160–78
  cancer treatment and 208
  caring for your hair 177–8
  changes to your hair 175–7
  facial-hair growth 177
  hair loss 176–7, 208, 287
  testosterone and 163–4
Harding, Prof Chris 67
hearing issues 53–4
the heart 99–101, 260–1, 271
  palpitations 54–5, 56
heartburn 55
heat therapy 47
herbal medicines 220
high-intensity interval training
  (HIIT) 269, 270
HIV 250
Holtom, Lucy 263–5
hormones 7–30
  after pregnancy 24–9
  during pregnancy 22–4
  endocrine system 9–10
  hormone deficiency 31–71, 136,
    139, 157
  hormones explained 9–11
  and mental health 136–59
  and weight gain 299, 300–1
  and your skin 163–4
  see also individual hormones and
    HRT
hot flushes 36, 40, 54, 55–7, 99,
  206
  treating 151, 214–15, 220, 264
HRT (hormone replacement therapy)
  53, 93–134, 352
  benefits of 96–101, 216

body-identical HRT 96, 97, 100,
  105–6, 114, 116, 117, 120
  and breast cancer 94, 117–19,
    120–1, 231, 232
  and breastfeeding 112–14
  and cancer 94, 103, 117–19,
    120–1, 215–19, 223–5, 231,
    232, 233
  and dementia risk 104–6
  and depression 141, 148–50, 159
  and diabetes 102–3
  and early menopause 186, 192–4,
    196–7, 216
  and hair loss 176–7
  healthcare and HRT experiences
    133–4
  and the heart 99–101
  how much to use 109, 110, 112
  and osteoporosis 97–8
  and the perimenopause 78, 100,
    107, 148
  positive impact of 121–2
  risks and side effects 110–12,
    117–21, 127
  and sleep 159
  stopping taking 115, 116
  treating skin complaints with 166,
    169
  vaginal hormones 129–33
  ways of administering 95, 96,
    108–9
  weight gain and 302
  what it is 95–6
  when to start taking 107, 115–16
  when to use 109–10
  see also oestrogen; progesterone;
    testosterone
human chorionic gonadotropin
  hormone (hCG) 23

human placental lactogen (hPL) 23
hyaluronic acid 163, 166
hypoactive sexual desire disorder
     (HSDD) 123, 124–6
hypothalamus 10, 23, 138
hysterectomy 121, 183, 218

immune cells, oestradiol and 11–12,
     97
immune system, boosting 306–7
inflammation 12, 57, 97, 103, 307
insulin 10, 102, 283, 292, 298, 300,
     302
iron 285–9
irritability 34, 36, 145, 147, 206–7

joint pain 57, 205, 208, 211, 298,
     300
Jones, Dr Wendy 112–14
jowls 170

Karim, Sarian 252
kefir, pink oats with 309–10
keratin 47, 177

Lalahy, Gaele 340–2
leptin 300–1
LGBTQ+ communities 247–9
libido 57–8, 96, 123, 124–6, 128–9,
     151, 209
lifestyle 21, 106, 120, 194, 214, 231
luteinising hormone (LH) 13

Macbeth, Dr Alison 225–7
McCall, Davina 354
marginalised communities 250–6
melatonin 10, 89
memory 11, 32
     see also brain fog

menopause: average age of 37, 76,
     77, 180
cancer and 202–35
definition of 37, 40
early menopause 76, 77, 97,
     179–201
effect on relationships 58–9
factors that won't influence 78
and family history 72–92
hormone deficiency 31–71
importance of inclusivity 236–56
symptoms 41–71, 147
menstrual cycle 20, 37, 42, 285
hormones 11, 12, 13
luteal phase 13, 14, 18
in perimenopause 39, 40
tracking 21
mental health 135–59, 178, 211
exercise and 270, 271
mindfulness and 143–7
sleep and 156–9
treatment options 140–50
metabolism 10, 301
microbiome 304–8
migraines 60–1, 275
mindfulness 143–7
mindfulness-based cognitive therapy
     (MBCT) 145
minority backgrounds 238–47
Mirena coil 78, 96, 121, 141, 194,
     195
moisturisers 172, 173–4
mood: cancer treatment and 206–7
gut health and 305–6
hormones and 13, 111, 123, 138–9
menopause and 60, 136, 138–59
mood-boosting berry smoothie 309
in perimenopause 21, 33, 39, 40,
     60, 136, 138–59

mood: cancer treatment and (*contd*)
  PMDD 18
  PMS 14, 15, 17, 21, 40
  postnatal 18, 24, 27, 113
  sleep and 157–8
Mosconi, Dr Lisa 104–6
motivation 158, 273, 281
mouths, dry 51–2
Muir, Kate 239–40, 351–2, 353–4
muscles 13, 57, 123

nails, brittle 47–8, 287
night sweats 33–4, 54, 55–7, 99,
    206, 214–15, 264
Norton, Dr Sally 302–4
nutrition and diet 214, 275–322
  calcium 10, 98, 212, 281–2, 283
  cancer treatment and 212
  carbohydrates and the glycaemic
    index 292–3
  and dementia risk 106
  eating your way to better health
    321–2
  fats 293–5
  fibre 291–2
  finding balance in your diet
    278–80
  gut health 304–20
  and hair loss 178
  iron 285–9
  and oral health 53
  plant oestrogens 289–90
  PMS and 21
  protein 290–1
  and tear production 50
  vitamin D 283–5
  weight gain and loss 298–304
Nwokolo, Dr Nneka 243–4

oats: calcium-rich Parmesan oatcakes
  318–19
  pink oats with kefir 309–10
obsessive-compulsive disorder (OCD)
  154–6
oestradiol 11–12, 97, 130, 132, 190,
  193–4, 223, 285
oestriol 11, 130, 132
oestrogen 11–12, 22, 45, 46, 78
  after pregnancy 25, 27, 113
  blood pressure and 99–100
  and bone health 98
  cancer and 216, 218, 222
  dementia and 105
  dizziness and 49
  early menopause 182–3, 192, 193
  effect of fluctuating levels of 38–9,
    42, 44–67, 138–9, 208, 300–1
  effect on blood vessels 49,
    99–100
  effect on mood 138–9
  and hair 176
  hearing issues 54
  HRT 95, 114, 119, 120, 127, 141,
    190
  and inflammation 12, 48, 57,
    103
  insulin production 102–3
  keratin production 47–8
  in menopause 42, 44–67
  mucus production 48
  'normal' ranges of 193–4
  and oral health 51
  and osteoporosis 197, 210, 217
  and pelvic-floor dysfunction 62,
    63, 67
  in perimenopause 38–9, 42,
    44–67
  and premature death 103

production of 10–11, 22, 189
selective oestrogen receptor
    modulators (SERM) 222–3
and sense of smell and taste 43
and skin 51, 163–4, 167, 169
and sleep 300
vaginal oestrogen 71, 114, 125,
    127, 130–3, 213, 229–30
oestrone 11, 299
Okoye, Dr Uchenna 52–3
omega-3 fatty acids 50, 293, 294
oral health 51–3
osteoporosis 12, 97–8, 116, 191,
    192, 197, 210, 216, 217, 281
ovaries 10–11, 22, 37, 39, 189, 204,
    231
  ovarian cancer 218
  premature ovarian insufficiency
    (POI) 180, 181–4, 185, 191–2
ovulation 11, 13, 39, 42
oxytocin 23, 24, 25, 301

pancreas 10, 292
parathyroid glands 10
Parkinson's disease 97, 104, 106
peer networks 255–6
pelvic-floor dysfunction 62–6, 69,
    265
People Arise Now 241
perimenopause 37–40
  changes to periods 39, 40, 44
  early signs of 36–7
  hormone deficiency 31–71
  HRT and 107, 148
  symptoms 21, 22, 33, 39–40,
    41–71, 147
  when and why it happens 37–9,
    180
periodontitis 51, 52, 53

periods 11, 38, 181, 187, 285, 286
  age of starting 78
  cancer treatment and 205, 206
  in menopause 43–4
  in perimenopause 37, 39, 40, 41,
    44
  premature ovarian insufficiency
    (POI) 182
pessaries 66, 130
Phipps, Dr Claire 241
phytoestrogens 289–90
pineal gland 10
pituitary gland 10, 12, 13, 23, 24
plant oestrogens 289–90
plaque 52–3
positive thoughts 152
postnatal depression (PND) 26–9,
    139, 152
pregabalin 215
pregnancy 11, 22–4, 43
premature ovarian insufficiency
    (POI) 180, 195–201, 204
  fertility and 194–201
  HRT and 192–4, 196–7
  investigation and diagnosis
    188–91
  long-term health risks 191–2
  treatment options 192–4
  what causes it 182–4
  what it is 181–2
premenstrual dysphoric disorder
    (PMDD) 18–20, 139, 152
premenstrual syndrome (PMS)
    14–18, 139, 152
  diagnosing 19–20
  in perimenopause 39–40
  seeking help for 20–2
  symptoms 15–16, 17–20, 21
  why it happens 14–15

prisons, menopause in 252–3
progesterone 25, 38, 42, 46, 49, 78
  early menopause and 192, 193,
    194
  effect on mood 138, 139
  HRT 95, 96, 111, 114, 141
  micronised progesterone 95, 96,
    110, 114, 119, 120, 141, 194
  pregnancy and 13, 22–3
  production of 10–11
progestogen 17, 95, 111, 119, 193,
  194
prolactin 24, 25
protein 290–1

racial differences 238–47
radiotherapy 183, 185, 204, 208
Rajpar, Dr Sajjad 171–5, 177–8
rapid eye movement (REM) sleep
  158
redness 167
relationships, hidden impact of
  menopause on 58–9
rice: comfort in a bowl 316–18
rosacea 167, 173

St John's wort 220
salads: ginger and mint slaw 314–16
  mint, avocado and bean salad
    313–14
  roasted beetroot and cauliflower
    salad 311–12
Samuel, Julia 81–4
sebum 163, 166
self-esteem 60, 125–6, 136, 147,
  161, 208
serotonin 60, 138, 214, 301
17 beta-oestradiol 95, 119, 192
sex: cancer treatment and 208–9

hypoactive sexual desire disorder
  (HSDD) 123, 124–6
libido 57–8, 96, 123, 124–6,
  128–9, 151
painful 57, 58, 71, 208, 209
testosterone HRT and 123, 124–6,
  128–9
Shades of Menopause 244
Simpson, Jane 63–6
skin 160–75, 208
  bruising, fragile skin and slow
    wound healing 169
  changes to 161–70
  common skin problems 166–8
  dry and itchy 50–1, 166–7, 178, 208
  effect of oestrogen on 163–4, 167,
    169
  redness and flushing 167
  skin routines 171–5
  spots and acne 164–5, 167–8,
    178
  sun damage 169, 170
  wrinkles, jowls and dull skin 170
slaw, ginger and mint 314–16
sleep 54, 123, 156–9, 162, 207
  and dementia risk 106
  exercise and 261–2, 264
  how to improve 158–9
  and hunger hormones 300–1
  sleep apnoea 157, 159
SMART goals 302–4
smell, altered sense of 43
smoking 47, 57, 98, 104, 119, 121,
  170
smoothie, mood-boosting berry
  309
social media 255–6
South Asian women 238–9, 240,
  245–6, 255, 284

Spector, Professor Tim 301–2
spots 167–8, 172, 178
strength training 270, 271
stress 55, 57, 61, 106, 144, 306
stress response 10, 299–300
sugary foods 53, 275, 281, 299
sun damage 169, 170
sunscreen 172, 173, 174
surgical menopause *see* early
    menopause
sweating, night 33–4, 54, 55–7, 99,
    206, 214–15, 264

tamoxifen 204, 206, 215, 220, 222–3
Tariq, Dr Shema 250
taste, altered sense of 43, 52
teenagers, broaching the menopause
    with 83, 86, 87–92, 355–6
teeth 51–3
testosterone 13, 45, 49, 99, 301
    early menopause 192, 194
    effect on mood 138, 139
    HRT 95, 96, 109, 112, 123–9, 148
    joint pain and 208, 300
    and libido 58, 96
    premature ovarian insufficiency
        (POI) 182, 183
    production of 11, 189
    and skin and hair 163–4
thyroid gland 10
tinnitus 53–4
Toby, Dr Martina 243–4
transdermal HRT 114, 119–20, 126
    skin patches 95, 106, 108–10,
        119–20, 129, 193
transgender people 248–9

unwinding 151–2
urinary problems 129–30, 208, 229

urinary incontinence 65, 213
urinary-tract infections (UTIs)
    66–7, 69, 213

vaginas 62, 71
    cancer treatment and
        genitourinary symptoms 208,
        229
    discharge 71, 111
    dryness 57, 58, 71, 114, 130, 208,
        209, 210, 213, 229, 298
    vaginal bleeding 44
    vaginal hormones 114, 125, 127,
        129–33, 213, 229–30
    vaginal prolapse 66
visceral fat 299, 302
vitamin D 98, 212, 283–5, 293
vulvovaginal atrophy 71

walking 145, 146, 260, 270, 271,
    274
Ward, Dr Hannah 20–2
Warsi, Baroness Sayeeda 332–3, 351
weight gain 281, 292, 293, 296,
    298–302
    exercise and 261
    gut health and 307
    vitamin D and 285
weight loss 302–4
Wicks, Joe 268–71
Wilson, Robert 117
womb cancer 218
women of colour 238–47
Women's Health Initiative (WHI)
    100, 103, 117–18
work 212, 323–48, 355
    advice for company CEOs 346–7
    advice for employers, managers
        and colleagues 339–43

employer's obligations 339–40
menopause policy at 335, 339, 346
rights in the workplace 334–5
supporting colleagues 347–8
telling your manager 335–7
wound healing 169
wrinkles 170

yoga 142, 143, 146, 258–9, 263–5, 266–7
yoghurt: mood-boosting berry smoothie 309
younger people, menopause in 179–201

Acknowledgements

Since being a very young girl, my ambition has always been to make people better and the privilege of being a doctor has enabled this to happen. My mission now is to improve the global health of women and I am determined to make a difference to as many people as possible. Preventing diseases is more important that treating diseases. Writing this book contributes to this mission.

However, I do not work in isolation. I have a rapidly growing team of healthcare professionals, mentors, colleagues, academics, scientists, educationalists, supporters, communication and PR experts, wellbeing gurus and friends who are working with me and enabling me to have a louder and more confident voice. More importantly they believe in what I am doing and they understand the sheer enormity of my work. There are too many to individually name but they know who they are, and I thank each and every one of them.

Misconceptions of people are not healthy or clever. The menopause has been wrongly portrayed and misunderstood for too long. Far too many perimenopausal and menopausal women have not been listened to for decades – often resulting in needless suffering. Every day there are misconceptions from others about my work, some who are very vocal in public, which is unfounded but relentless. The people that continue to support me and allow me to ignore these detractors and keep focused on my work.

The enthusiasm from the team at Yellow Kite has been unstoppable and I am so grateful to Kat Keogh who has worked incredibly closely with me throughout the creation of this book. I would like to thank Lauren Lunn-Farrow and The Expert Agency who helped secure the publication of this book.

I would be nothing without the strong foundations both of my parents gave me for the first 9 years of my life, and that my mother has given me since my father died in 1979. Every day I am thankful for the strong values that they instilled in me and I hope I have given these to my daughters Jess, Sophie and Lucy.

Above all I want to thank women – patients, social media followers and everyone else who knows about my work – without your support and encouragement, this book would never have been written.